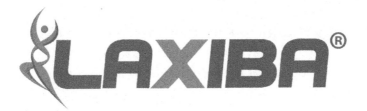

# THE LACTOSE NAVIGATOR

## The Standard for Lactose Intolerance

### 1. Edition

*The Nutrition Navigator Books Number Three*

## M.Sc. J. N. Stratbucker

LAXIBA

Houston

Copyright © 2017 by J. N. Stratbucker

ISBN 978-1-941978-75-7
Library of Congress Control Number 2016905803
Cover design by Mahmood Ali
Interior design by Katharina Maas and Mahmood Ali
Layout by Alexandra Krug
E-Mail of the author: John@Laxiba.com

Laxiba GmbH

Rotweinstrasse 12
53506 Rech
Germany

Victoria Botello
2840 Shadowbriar Drive Apt. 314
Houston, Texas, 77077, USA

**For companies and institutions:**
Are you interested in bulk orders? Visit us at: *https://laxiba.com*

The data set for the algorithmic ordained statements concerning lactose is from the University of Minnesota Nutrition Coordination Center 2014 Food and Nutrient Database. The reason to acquire the database license for this book were its high quality and scope based on international research. Statements regarding fructans and galactans result from six cited international studies. Nevertheless, the contents of the book bear no guarantee. Neither the author, publisher, any cited scientist nor the University of Minnesota is liable for personal injuries or physical or financial damage. Please note that the quantities of critical ingredients in the mentioned products, which are the foundation for the stated portion sizes, are relative and in part based on derivations. The serving sizes in this book are based on approximations of various details. The precise tolerable portion size of any product varies depending on its processing, country-specific composition, degree of maturity and cultivation.

*Manufactured in the United States of America*

FIRST EDITION

# Acknowledgments

Special thanks to M. Thor and the nutritional research team of the University of Minnesota, J. S. Barrett, J. R. Biesiekierski, P. R. Gibson, K. Liels, J. G. Muir, S. J. Shepherd, R. Rose and O. Rosella as well as the rest of the gastroenterology research team of the Monash University, all other cited scientists for their research, B. Hartmann of the Bundesministerium für Ernährung, Landwirtschaft und Verbraucherschutz, G.-W. von Rymon Lipinski of the Goethe University, and H. Zorn of the Justus Liebig University, for copyediting L. Gomes Domingues, F. Lang, C. R. Mundy, L. Popielinski, and M. Vastolo, for their feedback T. Albert, K. Bayer, U. Blendowske, D. Durchdewald, as well as my friends, especially C. Schlick and I. Kloppenburg, and all other contributors who enabled me to write this book in first place.

*To my friend Felix Lang for his reliability*

# Contents

# Preface

You just lately learned about your lactose sensitivity? Alternatively, are you well aware of your disease for many years? In each case, this book will help you, as it makes cooking and eating easy with its portion sizes in standard cooking measures as well as in gram and milliliter: scientifically proven and tested by readers like you. You may have tried out expensive medication or radical regimes like the FODMAP diet. Although the latter really works, it is unnecessarily strict. The aim of this book is to bring you more choice while you avoid your symptoms.

The book's information originates from intensive research and interviews with professors. The food tables in this book show you reliable serving sizes for foods concerning lactose intolerance. The design of the tables makes them easy to use. Moreover, they contain several specials. For example, you find the additionally tolerated amount per lactase enzyme capsule, you take, several ice cream brands, and the servings sizes for common lactose hideouts like certain sausages.

You do not have to avoid categorically all foods that contain lactose. It is enough to avoid eating more of them than you can stomach. By having as much choice as possible while preventing your symptoms, you increase your quality of life. How do you know how much your individual sensitivity allows you to eat? Quite simply, this book will tell you. Curious?

Then read on. In the first Chapter, you will learn about the diagnosis, backgrounds and consequences of the disease. Then in Chapter 2, you discover how to implement and keep the diet. You will also find a lot of advice there concerning healthy eating in general, recipes, hints of eating-out, strategies to stay motivated to stress management. Afterward, in Chapter 3 you will find the standard portion sizes for more than 1,000 products. Chapter 4 gives you even more advanced techniques to better adapt to your sensitivity. As I deal with an intolerance for a long time, I know about your need for clarity and practical advice. The focuses of my strategy are quality and suitability for daily use. I wholeheartedly wish you an ongoing success on your way to treat your symptoms and improve your quality of life!

*Note: Despite my aim to provide the highest quality, this book should not be the sole basis for any decision you make. Talk about any diet with your doctor before you begin to limit discomfort. You are responsible for your personal health, including how you choose to interpret data and specialists' advice. I cannot guarantee you a recovery. Several causes for your symptoms are possible—to find out more get THE IBS NAVIGATOR.*

# 1

# Information

## 1.1 Why you deserve this book

Congratulations: You take the initiative. By buying this book, you show your will to overcome your discomforts. If you bought this book, you know that a higher well-being is not only good for you but also everyone around you. Turn your back to the symptoms-grumbler. With the proper diet, you will feel healthier and stronger and enjoy more freedom!

Learn all you need to know about your disease, re-evaluate your personal story in that context and learn what you can do to live with it as best as possible. In addition, you find practical advice for a healthier diet in general on page 31 and on page 74 efficient methods to reduce stress, which often worsens your symptoms.

If you bought the book so you could learn to adapt to those in your life suffering from lactose intolerance, you would find out how in Chapter 2.5 and the one following it. Such behavior shows consideration for others that would make anyone glad to be a guest at your table!

That your nutrition affects your happiness is not a secret. It starts with your birth. A full and happy baby makes you happy too. The mother's milk provides the baby with the entire ingredients it needs and tolerates. As an adult, you choose the components of your nutrition yourself. Here it also holds that if you want to be satisfied, you need to eat the food your gut can handle.

Which diagnostic procedure should you have undergone? How does lactose affect me and how sensitive am I? How much can I eat of foods containing it without hurting myself? Which foods are free of lactose?

You get the answers for all of the mentioned questions. Explanations of the current scientific results and the most practical food tables for lactose intolerance on the market provide you with all you need to take proper action. On top of that, you find the cheat sheet for your wallet that enables you to adapt your diet even when eating out or going to the grocery store. Stop losing valuable energy to abdominal symptoms. Treat them right and start enjoying your life more instead, you deserve it!

# 1.2   Diagnostic check

A re abdominal pains, bloating, constipation, flatulence or diarrhea your ongoing companion? Without disrespect, we should find a way to get you a better spare time activity. Instead of accepting these discomforts, you should get the appropriate tools to free yourself from them as much as possible in order to spend more of your time enjoying the bright side of life.

The first thing you should do is to find out which of the potential triggers is the one that affects you. Just assuming you have a lactose intolerance is not enough. Going through all diagnostic procedures can take up half a year but will pay off. You will probably be able to get a handle on your symptoms and by using this book, you will also make sure to avoid unnecessary limitations concerning your diet , if you have indeed a lactose intolerance—otherwise get *THE IBS, THE FRUCTOSE* or *THE SORBITOL NAVIGATOR.*

To determine your profile, you should ask your local doctor to send you to an expert, a so-called gastroenterologist. Just the sound of this word might frighten your troublemakers. The specialist then first checks, whether your symptoms have a different cause than an intolerance. The diagnosis will include a **stool analysis**, an **ultrasonic check** and some camera shots inside your stomach to reject other reasons. These tests will allow the specialist to check whether there is an **abnormal bacterial colonization** of the small intestine. This migration may lead to false positives in uncovering an intolerance towards the **main triggers** covered in this book: **fructose, fructans, galactans, lactose,** and **sorbitol**. The next test looks for **celiac disease**, sensitivity towards gluten, which is an ingredient in grains. In people who have an untreated celiac disease, the tolerance test for the cube sorbitol is often positive, even if they can stomach it if they avoid gluten-containing foods. Following this, you should take a genetic test regarding **hereditary fructose** intolerance. Hereditary fructose intolerance is rare, but it is serious: the fructose test itself can be lethal to those with this disease.

You ruled out other potential causes, and the brats are probably trembling. Great, as now they are in for—what follows are checks regarding three of the mentioned main triggers. For the so-called breath test, you will take a high dose containing fructose, lactose or sorbitol on different days. If one of these passes through to your large intestine, due to suboptimal absorption by your body, gasses emerge. The doctors measure them to find out if you have an intolerance. When the amount of gas reaches a certain level, the diagnosis is an intolerance toward the respective trigger and have to adapt your diet accordingly. The threshold for a positive diagnosis for a lactose dilution (typically containing 25–50g) is usually 20ppm (parts per million, a concentration measure). This threshold also applies for fructose and sorbitol. The recommended breath test, however, is not available everywhere. In Chapter 2.2.1 you will learn about a substitute test, in case you have no access to the breath test.

Has the breath or substitute test shown that your body has enough capacity to handle even extreme amounts of a trigger? If so, you do not need to take any further attention to that trigger; its consumption will not cause you any harm — ignore the trigger: there is no point in taking unnecessary diets. If however the test shows that you have for example an intolerance towards lactose, you know which of the triggers you have to render harmless by limiting your consumption of foods in which it is present.

In general, do not accept a diagnosis without a test. If none of the tests comes to a conclusive result, you have an irritable bowel syndrome that is at least — for now — undefined. Irritable bowel just means that your gut reacts sensitively to various types of irritations such as gasses inside it — more on that in Chapter 1.4. The bowel is the final segment of your alimentary canal and the section where your symptoms come to show. Irritable bowel symptoms can be defined — if you have one of the before mentioned intolerances or undefined. If it is undefined, either, you did not take a test or it showed that you do not have an intolerance to one of the mentioned triggers. Note here that no breath-test is available for fructans and galactans as of now, and you will need to test your tolerance yourself, with my *IBS* book. In both cases, the symptoms are similar, because readily fermentable carbohydrates, a group that all triggers belong to, of some sort trigger the symptoms. Incidentally, for up to 90% of patients with an irritable bowel, an intolerance to one or more of the three breath-test-triggers mentioned above causes the symptoms.

If you suffer from irritable bowel symptoms, you are not alone: 20% of Americans have an intolerance, i.e., their enzyme worker team is too small for one or more of the three triggers that one tests with a breath test. Worldwide, 10–15% of all people suffer from undefined abdominal discomfort. About 20–30% of Europeans in general, 9% of the Dutch, 22% of the English, 25% of the Japanese and 44% of West Africans are affected. Concerning children, they should only take a diet under medical supervision. By the way, a lactose intolerance can only evolve at an age above five years. All younger children can stomach lactose.

It is also possible that a doctor finds that you are intolerant according to a breath test, but you do not feel symptoms. In such a case you may still want to keep the respective diet if you suffer from depressive moods, see Chapter 1.3.3.

## Summary

If you regularly suffer from abdominal discomfort, visit a specialist, a gastroenterologist. You may assume you have a lactose intolerance but only a specialist can rule out more severe diseases. Checks can take up to half a year. Many others share your fate; about 20% of Americans are affected. You are holding in your hands the key to fighting the symptoms!

# 1.3 Presentation of the triggers

**W**e depict lactose as cubes. Why? Just imagine having a big cube in your stomach. Not a good feeling. On the other hand, a cube can have a positive effect, too. Think of a sugar cube that provides a lot of energy. Likewise, lactose, being sugar related carbohydrates, provides you with energy, if your stomach makes uses it in that way.

## 1.3.1 How symptoms emerge

If you have an intolerance against lactose, your body only provides a few enzymes, which you can think of as workers making sure your body uses the cube for energy. Few workers mean that if you eat too much of foods that contain lactose cubes, many remain unused by your body and arrive at your large intestine. Now, two processes are responsible for the symptoms: osmosis and fermentation. To understand osmosis, let us imagine two equal fish bowls connected by an underwater tube.

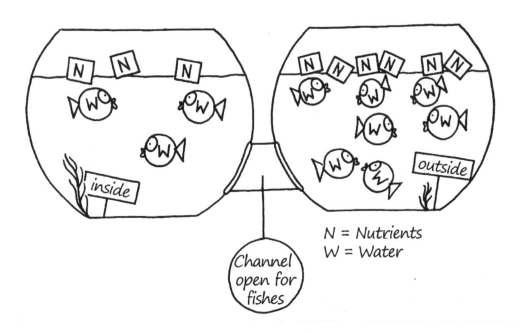

The glass on the left represents the inside of the bowel and the one on the right for the outside of it. The fishes represent water (W), and their food are either nutrient (N) or lactose cubes that arrive at the inside of the bowel (L). The channel enables fishes to switch between the bowls. Thus, they always swim to the glass that contains more food. Usually, this would be the outside of the intestine. Thereby, the body detracts the water from the foods—which is a good.

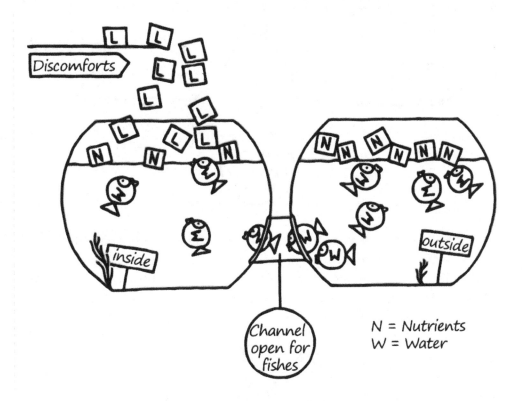

However, if you more of foods containing lactose than your enzyme workers can handle, lactose cubes arrive at the inside of the bowel. Hence, suddenly there is more food in the left fish bowl.

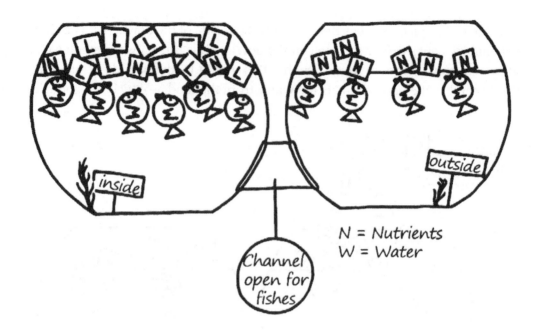

N = Nutrients
W = Water

As the intestinal wall, here represented by the channel, is only partially permeable, the fishes can swim through it, unlike the food. Therefore, some fishes now switch sides and scrimmage on the left. Their movement to the left means that with the cubes water arrives inside the intestine and you suffer from diarrhea.

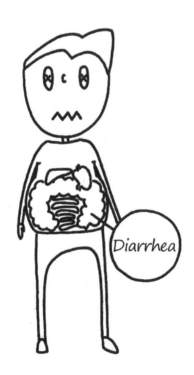

Now you know about osmosis. What causes fermentation?

As you know, you have bacteria inside your bowel, which is normal and that way for any healthy person. The issue is that these bacteria love sweets. Hence, if a lactose cube arrives at the large intestine, they do not falter and immediately consume it to help themselves to some energy.

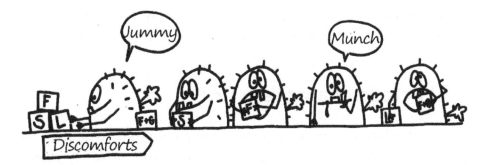

Unfortunately, though, the bacteria are less efficient at consuming the lactose cubes than our body is. When bacteria use the lactose cubes, gas emerges.

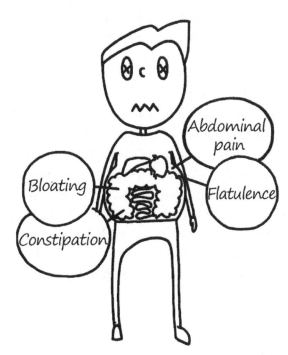

The gas either leaves as bloating or amounts and causes an uncomfortable flatulence. If the pressure increases in some regions of the intestines, this can cause deposits—constipation. If the gas enters the small intestine, it causes, even more, turmoil: it hinders some of the enzymes—the body's cube workers—from doing their job. That is because the workers mainly sit on the gut wall and the gas reduces its contact to the stool. However, what about the treatment with a diet? In general, it is important for your health to have a diverse diet. The FOD-MAP approach, which you may have heard of, aims at reducing the fermentation and osmosis by lowering the consumption of all potential triggers at once. With the lactose standard treatment of this book, you take a more precise aim to give you more freedom concerning your food choice. With it, you only avoid lactose, as described in the diagnosis check. First, you should get to know it, though.

## 1.3.2   Lactose characteristics

Another name for lactose is milk sugar as it is present primarily in milk and dairy products. Unfortunately, milk sugar is also included in many convenience foods, where you would not expect it to be. Bologna, coating, sauce and even medicine may contain it. Pure milk tends to have the highest share while some dry cheese, like cheddar, is nearly free of it. Luckily, you are still able to stomach a limited amount of lactose despite having a lactose intolerance and there are enzyme capsules to help you increase that amount further. Moreover, nowadays, there are a lot of lactose freed or milk replacement products such as rice milk or soymilk. Be careful though with soymilk. It contains the triggers fructans and galactans and may lead you out of the frying pan into the fire. Rice milk, on the contrary, is also free of that and thus the better alternative.

At the start of your life, lactose is irreplaceable: All small children are dependent on lactose and can tolerate it. At the end of the fifth year, the earliest a lactose intolerance can evolve. About 5 to 17 % of the light-skinned and 50 to 100 % of the rest of the population are affected. Still, not all of them suffer from symptoms at the same level. Most patients tolerate small amounts of lactose and not all of them suffer from a sensitive bowel. Nevertheless, why do some humans react to lactose with symptoms and other do not? How do the symptoms evolve? The following illustrations will show it to you.

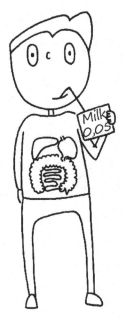

*Man with lactose intolerance*

Milk contains lactose by nature: 100 mL contain round about 5g of it. In the image, you can see John. Due to his lactose intolerance, he only has a few sips of milk, about 50 mL in total. He knows that he only has a few enzymes to degrade lactose in the small intestine.

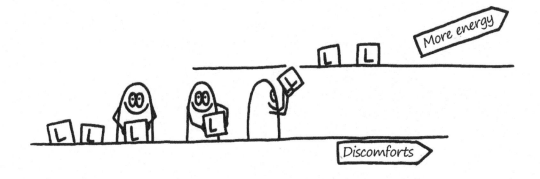

His enzymes, workers, are fine with handling the amount of lactose contained in the 50 mL—in case that is it for this meal. When our body assimilates the lactose (L) by the work of the enzymes, it provides us with energy. The symptoms stay away and everything goes swimmingly.

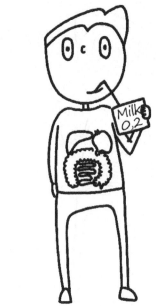

Man <u>with</u> Lactose intolerance

However, now John forgets that his team of lactose enzymes is easy to count. He now drinks a whole pack of milk containing 200 mL and has them work up a sweat.

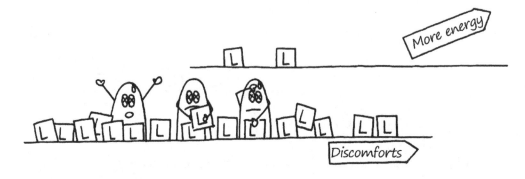

His enzymes cannot handle the load. The sudden flow of lactose is too much for them, and therefore, a lot of it remains on the "conveyor belt". This unprocessed lactose then reaches the large intestine and there it triggers symptoms.

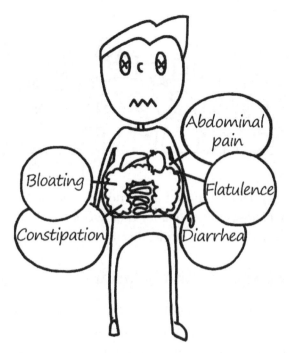

Some hours after the consumption he gets the bill: abdominal pain, bloating, diarrhea and flatulence.

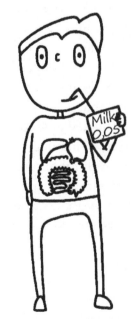

Man _without_ lactose intolerance

It is different with Chris, who is also drinking 200 mL.

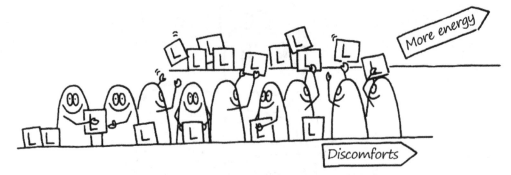

Chris does not have a lactose intolerance and thus has a far bigger team from the start. His many lactose-enzyme labor men work hand in hand are handling the amount quickly and can only smile about their groaning comrades.

## The influence of fructans and galactans

In a study, scientists were surprised to find that people suffering from a lactose intolerance were reacting with symptoms to a lactose-free test milk. The reason for this, which I implied is that although the lactose-free milk did not contain lactose, it did still contain other readily fermented (potentially symptom-triggering) carbohydrates, galactans. How much of the latter is contained in milk, depends on the race, month and the lactation period of the animals. The highest average amount is contained in cow milk with 0.137g/100 mL, followed by goat milk with 0.117g/100 mL. Per gram lactose, you can thus add 0.03g to galactans. It thus takes longer to reach the threshold of your sensitivity. However, in combination with other foods like cereals, they can be just the amount that takes it from tolerated to symptoms. That may also be the explanation for the continuing symptoms of some, who consciously avoid lactose, still do not manage to get rid of their discomforts to a satisfying degree.

For some, the intestine reacts even more sensitive to fructans and galactans than towards lactose. Are you one of these unlucky fellows—are you unsatisfied with the symptom reduction by the lactose diet? If so, I recommend you buy *THE IBS NAVIGATOR* and try the fructan and galactan diet.

## Your personal sensitivity

If you find that you would rather like to avoid osmosis and fermentation in this context, then batten down the hatches! Make sure that no lactose arrives at your large intestine. Reduce your lactose consumption to the amount that your enzymes can handle. The level that you should not top, in order not to have your enzymes lose the game is usually 10g of lactose per day, which equals about 3.3g per meal. With the standard amounts in the nutrition tables at the end of this book, you eat up to 3g of lactose per meal. Here you see how much you can eat of what. By the way, the amount of lactose that medicine contains, which you take in orally, is usually so small that you should be able to tolerate it if you avoid the consumption of other lactose-containing foods during the treatment.

## Calcium

If you limit your consumption of milk products, it is important that you take in calcium in alternative ways, as your body needs it. Adults below 50 should take about 1,000mg per day (teenagers even 1,300mg) and women above 50 as well as men above 60, 1,200mg. You can take in calcium via some lactose free milk or milk replacement products, protein powders (1,200mg per 100g), Cheddar cheese, (721mg per 100g), almonds (236mg per 100g), anchovy and salmon (240mg per 100g), spinach in all variants (210mg per 100g) and figs (162g per 100g) or calcium pills. In case you use supplements, try to find some that are lactose-free.

## Lactase enzyme capsules

As you can expect to be able to stomach 3g of lactose per meal, it only makes sense to take a capsule if you exceed this amount. For the lactose enzymes you take to have an effect, they have to arrive at the small intestine, where they go to work. There is no use in taking them if the enzymes reach the stomach un-protected. The gastric acid there would only destroy them. Gastric acid resistant capsules are suited best for bringing the enzymes safely to their workplace. By the way, they ought to arrive at the same time that lactose does for an optimal effect. A study showed that the most effective capsule, containing 12,000 FCC[1], was only able to neutralize 2.7g of lactose. Thus, to cover a 237 mL, after sub-tracting the 3g per meal, you still need at least four capsules.

If you are nostalgically thinking of your math class, which you spent freshly in love or crapulous rather below than on you chair and already, have the: "If only I had paid more attention" on your mind: No worries! You do not have to be a master in mental arithmetic to apply this knowledge. You not only find the tolerated amounts but also the additionally tolerated amount per capsules esti-mated for you in the food tables of this book.

---

[1] *Food Chemical Codex, measurement unit for enzymes.*

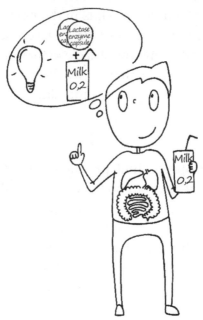

Man <u>with</u> lactose intolerance

John has just gotten smarter. Once more, he wants to drink a whole 200 mL box of milk. As he knows that this amount will cause him an abdominal pain without preparations, he takes four high-dose lactase capsules (12,000 FCC) in advance.

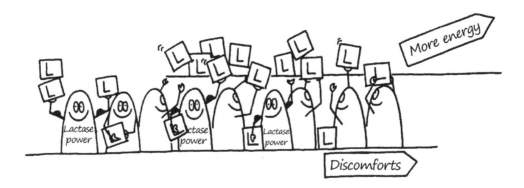

His enzymes thus receive dynamic support and can tackle the incoming amount of lactose. Thereby, John is free from symptoms.

## Lactose-free milk (replacement) products

Many lactose freed dairy products as well as milk replacement products, such as soy or rice milk are available in stores. These offer you the opportunity to look at the tables in this book, as you will find many products, such as cheese, of which you can consume quite a lot.

Hint: in case you have a fructans and galactans sensitivity, you should prefer rice to soymilk products, as it is free of it.

# 1.3.3   Consequences of a lactose intolerance

## Physical effects

You are already familiar with the immediate effects of an untreated fructose intolerance: abdominal pain, bloating, diarrhea and flatulence. These alone are certainly enough to have you take action. However, indirectly they can also lead to lower lust, reduced social contacts, lower empathy and less vitality in general. Hence, not handling your intolerance lowers your quality of life. It is not so surprising that this also affects your days off work. A study, done in the USA and the Netherlands, shows that on average people with an untreated intolerance take about twice as many sick leaves from school or work than do their peers. Luckily, you can do something about that. You can recapture your well-being by learning how to adapt your diet to your capacity to absorb lactose. Ideally, you only limit your nutrition as far as is necessary—a certain amount of lactose is usually even tolerable if you are intolerant towards lactose. My aim is to make this as easy as possible for you.

## Depression

Scientists have found that there is a causal relation between having an untreated intolerance and increased depression scores. The reason for this is a reduced prevalence of a neurotransmitter, serotonin, in case lactose arrives at the large intestine. Serotonin elevates one's mood. The body produces it from trypto-phan, which it derives from food. Presumably, at least, lactose that passes the small intestine—remains on the belt—merges with tryptophan to form a non-absorbable substance. This reaction reduces the amount of available tryptophan and causes the body to produce less serotonin. Hence, lactose that arrives at the large intestine hinders the body's ability to let positive feelings emerge. In an experiment in which patients lowered their trigger consumption, depression scores normalized for most participants. Keeping the consumption limits that apply to you when choosing your portion sizes can improve your mood (your serotonin metabolism) because fewer lactose arrives at the large intestine. Extra discipline is required to maintain the portion thresholds in cases of depression, however, as a lack of high spirits (tryptophan) can foster the hunger for sweets. Now, candies often contain lactose. If an intolerance is present, the intake of lactose containing sweets further lowers one's mood, creating a vicious circle. You can find out how much you can eat for many foods in the lists in Chapter 3. Even if you are not depressed, please remember that in the presence of a dysfunctional metabolism, depression can result from consuming too much of foods that contain problematic ingredients. Affected people should always seek help rather than trying to counter these effects through sheer willpower and bear in mind that they can and should do something about ongoing feelings of sadness, little personal power, and low energy.

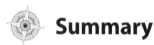 ## Summary

**Fructans, galactans and lactose are carbohydrates that bacteria ferment if they reach the large intestine. In that case, they cause various abdominal symptoms. Many foods contain lactose. In case of a lactose intolerance, you have too few enzyme workers making sure your body uses lactose to gain energy before it can reach the large intestine. You treat your symptoms by limiting your consumption of lactose to the capacity of your enzyme workers. To do so, you eat according to the tables in the third Chapter showing you the tolerated amount per meal. Our tables enable you to reduce the amount of lactose you eat so far that you avoid your symptoms while enjoying as much freedom as is possible concerning your choice of foods.**

# 1.4   Background of an irritable bowel

Suffering from lactose intolerance symptoms is like having a sensitive colon. Like a notorious diva, the intestine shows a lack of robustness and an oversensitivity. It will not allow tampering with, reacts disappointed and offended when ignored by someone that offers her unfitting food. In the case of stress, she pipes up even more vehemently. Many people are carrying such a diva around with them, which repeatedly makes her demands known.

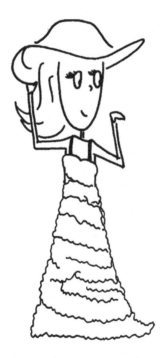

By the way, the exact causes of the diva's show up are unknown. An assumption is that people living in regions with less sunlight developed the ability to use lactose after childhood because drinking milk enabled them a better supply with some vitamins, which the body generates when exposed to the sun. In any case, it has nothing to do with the character. Having a diva-tummy not at all means having a diva-like congeniality.

# 1.5 Abdominal discomfort in kids

In general, abdominal discomforts of your child can have a variety of reasons. A lactose intolerance will not occur before the age of five. Other potential triggers of abdominal pain, bloating and diarrhea in children are fructose and sorbitol: Children ages 14 to 58 months drank 250 mL of apple juice in a study. Afterward, all children who suffered from chronic diarrhea, as well as 65.5% of the healthy children, tested positive for malabsorption-symptoms. Avoiding apple juice led to recovery for **all** of the children. This result corresponds with other research that shows that many children suffer from diarrhea and abdominal pain if they drink too much fruit juice. Liquids that contain high levels of sorbitol are often the trigger. You should give your child a maximum of 10 mL juice per kilogram of body weight. Moreover, you should avoid giving them fruit juices that contain sorbitol or high amounts of free fructose, like apple or peach juice.

# 2

## STRATEGY

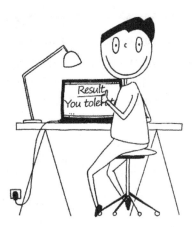

## 2.1　A gut's change management

No employee likes to stay at a company that always overstrains him. Equally unsatisfactory is to work at a place where one gets the feeling that one does not contribute at all. The typical consequences of both extremes: lack of motivation, an increase in the number of sick leaves up to an incapacity to work at the place anymore. What does that have to do with you? Quite simply: what goes in the professional environment, applies to your bowel as well. Hence, you should strive to work with your enzymes (conveyor-belt workers) in a team instead of over- or under-straining them. Show your leadership qualities and make your staff your motivated allies instead of waiting for them to come to you with their complaints!

How you can get that done, you will find out in this book. Did you ever want to rely on a master plan? If that is so, you will like what follows. According to the following plan, you will first determine the status quo of your symptoms. The next step is to keep a lactose diet for three weeks. At the end you determine, whether your symptoms have improved. If so, you can find out whether you can stomach more than the standard amounts—better adapt to the capacity of your workers. If your symptoms did not improve to your satisfaction, work on your stress management according to Chapter 2.8 or get *THE IBS NAVIGATOR* to search for alternative triggers.

## 2.1.1  Signpost

| Status-quo-check: | Introduction diet: | Efficiency check: | Adaption: |
|---|---|---|---|
| Note down your symptoms for four days **before** the diet | Keep the the lactose diet according to the food tables in Chapter 3. | Note down your symptoms on the last four days of your introductory diet to determine if the diet worked. If not, check alternative causes. | Sensitivity check to find out if you can tolerate more than the standard serving sizes. |

## 2.1.2 Roadmap

| Step | Action | Target |
|------|--------|--------|
| **Duty** <br> **1** | **Status-quo-check** <br> Fill out the symptom test sheet <br> Duration: 4 days | Determining your status quo: Which symptoms do you have, and how severe are they? |
| **Optional** <br> **2** | **Breath tests at a specialist** <br> Duration: 4 days | As you bought this book, you have either already taken it or done the substitute test in *THE IBS NAVIGATOR*. Otherwise, you can take the introductory diet to find out if the lactose diet works for you but it is more advisable to check for alternative triggers as well and for that, you need the book or a breath test. |
| **Duty** <br> **3** | **Introductory diet and efficiency check with symptom test sheet** <br> Symptom tracking during the last four days of the diet. <br> Duration of the diet: <br> three weeks | You keep the lactose diet with the Chapter 3 tables and fill out the symptom test sheet. Did the diet lower your symptoms satisfactory? <br><br> **Yes)** Continue with step four. <br><br> **No)** Retry with half the amounts. Otherwise, work on the stress management chapter or follow the introductory diet for the alternative triggers fructans and galactans in *THE IBS NAVIGATOR*. |
| **Optional** <br> **4** | **Sensitivity-level-test** <br> Duration: <br> ~½ month | Enabling you a diet that is as varied as possible while reducing your symptoms is possible by determining your sensitivity level, see Chapter 4. |

The goal of the overall strategy is to determine how much you tolerate without causing "the diva" to protest. The first step towards that goal it to determine the status quo, the severity of your symptoms, before changing your diet. The reason for this is that this is the only way to check, whether the diet has an effect.

To do so, note down your discomforts in a copy of the following symptom test sheet. **Make sure to keep your symptom test sheets in a folder.** The days at which you note down your symptoms should be average to you. Neither a day on which you sickly vegetated in your bed nor one on which you celebrated the stag party of your best friend or had to master a difficult test count. If you are uncertain about whether it was an average day, cross it out. **Important: This also holds true for all of the subsequent tests. If you are in doubt as to whether the day was "normal," i.e. no circumstances distorted the symptoms, repeat the test to get a more reliable result.** On the days where you track your symptoms, always carry a copy of the symptom test sheet with you. Ideally, you should fill it out right after your main meals, e.g., at 7 am, 1 pm and 7 pm. After the four days of your status quo check, you should also be able to classify the type of stool you usually have. Depending on whether you have constipation, diarrhea or a mix of both, you are an IBS-C, IBS-D or IBS-M type. If you have neither constipation nor diarrhea, your IBS type is unclassified. Take that information with you when you visit the doctor. After tracking your symptoms for four days, follow the introductory diet. That means you keep a diet according to the tables in Chapter 3. In the last week, you then fill out the symptom test sheet to determine the diet's effectiveness. If keeping the diet leads to an improvement of your well-being that you are satisfied with, you should stick to it. You can read how to assess the test sheets more professionally than just laying the one before next to the one after the diet in Chapter 4.3. You can use the efficiency-check-symptom-sheet later as a reference for the sensitivity-level-test, if you decide to take it—it is also included in the advanced techniques-Chapter 4. With the latter, you can adjust to your enzyme worker's capacities to handle lactose.

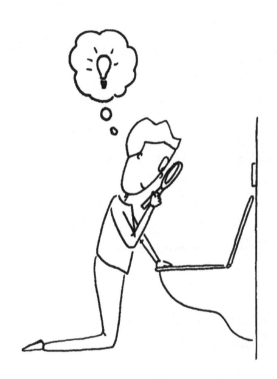

## Stool types after Bristol

| | | |
|---|---|---|
| | Separate hard lumps, like nuts (hard to pass) | **Type** A: Constipation<br><br>**Value** 4 |
| | Sausage-shaped but lumpy | **Type** B: Constipation<br><br>Value 2 |
| | Like a sausage but with cracks on the surface | **Type** C: normal<br><br>**Value** 1 |
| | Like a sausage or snake, smooth and soft | **Type** D: normal<br><br>**Value** 1 |
| | Soft blobs with clear-cut edges | **Type** E: Diarrhea<br><br>**Value** 2 |
| | Fluffy pieces with ragged edges, a mushy stool | **Type** F: Diarrhea<br><br>**Value** 4 |
| | Watery, no solid pieces; **entirely liquid** | **Type** G: Diarrhea<br><br>**Value** 5 |

(Based on Lewis & Heaton, 1997; Thompson, 2006)

Types 3 and 4 are the norm. The farther away your type is from these two, the worse your ailments.

# 2.1.3  Symptom test sheet

Note down your stool type in the morning ✹, afternoon ☀, and evening ☾ and your stool value from 1 to 5 (see page 26) as well as the number of times you visited the toilet to estimate the stool grade by multiplying the numbers. Also, evaluate bloating and pain from 1 to 5 according to the following scale:

1  No discomfort, like someone without symptoms
2  Hardly any discomfort relative to someone without symptoms
3  Medium discomfort relative to someone without symptoms
4  Severe discomfort relative to someone without symptoms
5  Very severe discomfort relative to someone without symptoms

**Test:**_____ **End date:**_____

For each test, you need copies of this page!

| | | Type/ Value | Defecation count | | Stool grade | + | Bloating grade | + | Pain grade | = B | |
|---|---|---|---|---|---|---|---|---|---|---|---|
| **Day 1 prior** | ✹ | | x | = | | | | | | | **TEST DAY** |
| | ☀ | | x | =(+) | | + | | + | | | |
| | ☾ | | x | =(+) | | + | | + | | | |
| | | The day's sum | A = | | | = | | = | | | |
| **Day 2 prior** | ✹ | | x | = | | | | | | | **Day 1 after** |
| | ☀ | | x | =(+) | | + | | + | | | |
| | ☾ | | x | =(+) | | + | | + | | | |
| | | The day's sum | A = | | | = | | = | | | |
| **Day 3 prior** | ✹ | | x | = | | | | | | | **Day 2 after** |
| | ☀ | | x | =(+) | | + | | + | | | |
| | ☾ | | x | =(+) | | + | | + | | | |
| | | The day's sum | A = | | | = | | = | | | |
| **Day 4 prior)** | ✹ | | x | = | | | | | | | **Day 3 after** |
| | ☀ | | x | =(+) | | + | | + | | | |
| | ☾ | | x | =(+) | | + | | + | | | |
| | | The day's sum | A = | | | = | | = | | | |

# Example: The four status quo (1.)/Level (2.) check days

Note down your stool type in the morning 🐓, afternoon ☀, and evening ☾ and your stool value from 1 to 5 (see page 26) as well as the number of times you visited the toilet to estimate the stool grade by multiplying the numbers. Also, evaluate bloating and pain from 1 to 5 according to the following scale:

1 No discomfort, like someone without symptoms
2 Hardly any discomfort relative to someone without symptoms
3 Medium discomfort relative to someone without symptoms
4 Severe discomfort relative to someone without symptoms
5 Very severe discomfort relative to someone without symptoms

**Test:**_____ **End date:**_____

For each test, you need copies of this page!

| | | Type/ Value | Defecation count | | Stool grade | Bloating grade | Pain grade | |
|---|---|---|---|---|---|---|---|---|
| **Day 1 prior** | 🐓 | E 2 | x 2 | = | 4 | 2 | 2 | **TEST DAY** |
| | ☀ | F 4 | x 2 | =(+) | 8 | + 2 | + 3 | |
| | ☾ | E 2 | x 2 | =(+) | 4 | + 3 | + 2 | |
| | | | The day's sum | = | 16 | = 7 | = 7 | |
| **Day 2 prior** | 🐓 | F 4 | x 2 | = | 8 | 2 | 3 | **Day 1 after** |
| | ☀ | E 2 | x 1 | =(+) | 2 | + 3 | + 4 | |
| | ☾ | F 4 | x 1 | =(+) | 4 | + 2 | + 2 | |
| | | | The day's sum | = | 14 | = 7 | = 9 | |
| **Day 3 prior** | 🐓 | E 2 | x 1 | = | 2 | 2 | 3 | **Day 2 after** |
| | ☀ | F 4 | x 2 | =(+) | 8 | + 2 | + 4 | |
| | ☾ | E 2 | x 1 | =(+) | 2 | + 3 | + 5 | |
| | | | The day's sum | = | 12 | = 7 | = 12 | |
| **Day 4 prior)** | 🐓 | F 4 | x 1 | = | 4 | 2 | 2 | **Day 3 after** |
| | ☀ | E 2 | x 1 | =(+) | 2 | + 2 | + 2 | |
| | ☾ | F 4 | x 2 | =(+) | 8 | + 3 | + 3 | |
| | | | The day's sum | = | 14 | = 7 | = 7 | |

## Example: The four efficiency check days

Note down your stool type in the morning 🐓, afternoon ☀, and evening ☾ and your stool value from 1 to 5 (see page 26) as well as the number of times you visited the toilet to estimate the stool grade by multiplying the numbers. Also, evaluate bloating and pain from 1 to 5 according to the following scale:

1  No discomfort, like someone without symptoms
2  Hardly any discomfort relative to someone without symptoms
3  Medium discomfort relative to someone without symptoms
4  Severe discomfort relative to someone without symptoms
5  Very severe discomfort relative to someone without symptoms

**Test:**_____ **End date:**_____

For each test, you need copies of this page!

| | | Type/ Value | Defecation count | Stool grade | Bloating grade | Pain grade | |
|---|---|---|---|---|---|---|---|
| **Day 1 prior** | 🐓 | - | x 0 | = 0 | 1 | 1 | **TEST DAY** |
| | ☀ | E 2 | x 1 | =(+) 2 | + 1 | + 1 | |
| | ☾ | D 1 | x 1 | =(+) 1 | + 1 | + 1 | |
| | | | The day's sum | = 3 | = 3 | = 3 | |
| **Day 2 prior** | 🐓 | D 1 | x 1 | = 1 | 1 | 1 | **Day 1 after** |
| | ☀ | - | x 0 | =(+) 0 | + 1 | + 1 | |
| | ☾ | D 1 | x 1 | =(+) 1 | + 1 | + 1 | |
| | | | The day's sum | = 2 | = 3 | = 3 | |
| **Day 3 prior** | 🐓 | D 1 | x 1 | = 1 | 1 | 1 | **Day 2 after** |
| | ☀ | - | x 0 | =(+) 0 | + 2 | + 2 | |
| | ☾ | E 2 | x 1 | =(+) 2 | + 1 | + 1 | |
| | | | The day's sum | = 3 | = 4 | = 4 | |
| **Day 4 prior)** | 🐓 | - | x 0 | = 0 | 1 | 1 | **Day 3 after** |
| | ☀ | D 1 | x 1 | =(+) 1 | + 1 | + 1 | |
| | ☾ | D 1 | x 1 | =(+) 1 | + 1 | + 1 | |
| | | | The day's sum | = 2 | = 3 | = 3 | |

# 2.1.4 Keeping your balance

Now, you know if the diet provides you benefits and maybe even, how sensitive you are. Still, aside from avoiding the consumption of too much of your trigger, you should also learn some generally advisable nutrition principles.

| | | |
|---|---|---|
| 1 | Eat a rich variety of foods, i.e., something different each day and with lots of natural ingredients. Eat with a relaxed posture. | 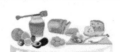 |
| 2 | Take care of your supply of fiber, e.g., by eating potatoes, flax seeds, lentils, nuts. |  |
| 3 | Ingest five portions of vegetables (ideally dark green, red or orange) and fruit. | 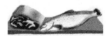 5/day |
| 4 | Have some reduced-fat milk products like reduced-fat milk, yogurt or cheese every day. |  |
| 5 | One or two times a week, eat fish and eggs, as well as 300–600g of low-fat meat, ideally poultry. |  |
| 6 | Use vegetable oils if possible, like canola oil, and fats. |  |
| 7 | Reduce your consumption of salt and sugar. |  |
| 8 | Drink at least 1.5 liters of non-alcoholic drinks per day. Best are unsweetened beverages and water. Drink alcohol moderately or avoid it entirely. |  |
| 9 | Preferably, cook fresh and at lower temperatures to reduce nutrient leaching. |  |
| + | Stay fit: exercise regularly. |  |

## Potential compensation needs due to your diet

In the following, you will learn that due to short-chained fatty acids you should not entirely dispense milk products even if you are of being intolerant towards lactose. As a guideline for your nutrition, find the recommended daily amounts in respective bowls.

## Proteins

**Proteins**
**0.66g/kg**

One needs 0.66g of protein per kilogram of body weight per day. You can ensure your protein supply by consuming the following products. The rough amount of proteins per portion is shown in parenthesis: 85g meat (28g protein), 85g fish (26g), 150 mL instant coffee with or without caffeine (18g, but standard espresso contains only 0.3g), 200 mL whole milk with added vitamin D (15g), 200 mL whole milk or fat-free milk without additives (6g), 85g corn or wild rice (12g), 90g kidney beans (18g), 140g pasta (15g), 90g soybeans (14g), a medium-sized egg (7.5g), 90g lentils (8g), 110g potatoes (4g), 25g nuts, especially peanuts, peanut butter and almonds (5g), a slice of whole grain bread (5g), 25g cheese (4g), a slice of rice bread (3.5g), 30g cereal (3g), 24g rice bran (3g), 25g dark chocolate (2g) and 50g couscous (1.5g). You may notice that maintaining a supply of protein is rather easy. Vegetarians, however, should plan their protein intake consciously.

## Short-chained fatty acids

**S.-c. fatty acids**
**1.2/1.3g/day**

Short-chain fatty acids are important energy suppliers. Foods that are particularly rich in short-chain fatty acids include (fatty acids per portion without triglycerides in parenthesis): 10g butter (0.5g), 25g goat's cheese (0.5g), 25g gouda, Swiss cheese, cheddar or Roquefort (0.4g), 50g mozzarella (0.3g), 47g M&M's® (0.3g), 25g blue cheese (0.25g), 20 mL coconut oil (0.2g), 50g coconut meat (0.18g), 150g French fries (0.13g) or 20 mL palm kernel oil (0.08g).

As I said, I recommend the consumption of milk products in tolerable amounts, according to the tables in Chapter 3. Remember that your enzyme-workers should not be undertrained either and that these products are very rich concerning these fatty acids.

Experts recommend that short-chain fatty acids amount to 1/60 of the daily amount of consumed fats, which ought to be 70g for women and 80g for men. Thus, the required minimum daily intake is 1.2g per day for females and 1.3g for males. With a lactose intolerance, you can reach this amount easily by eating three slices of cheddar, a cheese that contains hardly any lactose. If you are a vegan, reaching the target is a challenge.

## Omega 3 fatty acids

Now talking about fatty acids let me explain another type, which is not impaired by the diet but at times enters the public discussions, omega 3 fatty acids. Women should take in 6.1g of the omega 3 fatty acid known as alpha-linolenic acid, or ALA while men should take in 7g. Alternatively, maintaining a 2:1 proportion of omega 6 to omega 3 will lead to an intake of up to 9.6g per day for women and 11g for men. ALA fatty acids have a positive effect on your cardiovascular system. The following foods contain high levels (rough ALA amount per portion in parenthesis): 200g fish (4g), 20 mL flaxseed oil (10.5g) for which the consumed amount should be below 100 mL per day (flaxseeds themselves contain 25% oil and thus 24g of flaxseeds, at least 3g; however, during pregnancy you should avoid both as it can harm your baby), 20 mL canola oil (1.8g), 20 mL mayonnaise (1g), 20 mL soy oil (0.8g), 100g wheat crackers (0.8g), 70g French fries (0.3g), 16g peanut butter with omega 3 (0.5g), 25g walnuts (0.5g), 10g butter (0.3g) and 10g margarine (0.3g). The data sheds a positive light on the fiber Strategy A as described in the following. You can reach the target amount of 7g for men just by consuming 1 tbsp. flaxseed oil per day. Alternatively, you can arrive at 6g, for example, by eating three portions of salad with 20 mL of canola oil each and a slice of bread with omega 3 peanut butter. Apart from ALA, EPA (eicosapentaenoic acid) and DHA (docosahexaenoic acid) are also essential. Your daily intake of EPA should be 250mg and of DHA, 500mg. If you eat fish at any time during the week, you will usually have covered your need. Krill or fish oil capsules containing these amounts are an alternative.

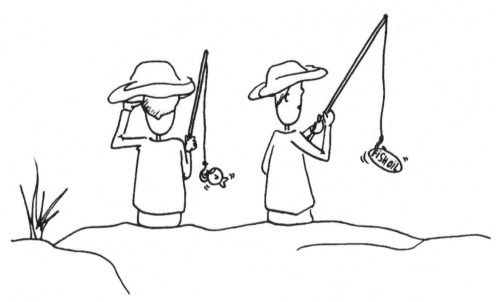

##  Summary

**As part of the strategy, you first note down your symptoms before doing anything. Then you start the introductory diet. For it, you reduce the consumption of lactose. The aim is to check whether the diet lowers your symptoms after all. So, fill out the symptom-test-sheet before starting the diet. Then follow the diet according to the tables in Chapter 3 for three weeks and fill out the test-sheet once more for the last four days. If you are feeling better now, you can also determine your precise sensitivity level; see Chapter 4. If you still have symptoms, follow steps two and three as described on the next page.**

### Make sure you keep a balanced diet:

Drink least 1.5 liters of water per day and exercise regularly. Possibly, your diet requires you to compensate with regard to the following ingredients:

**Proteins:** For example, by eating fish, meat, eggs rice or rice bran.

**Short-chain fatty acids:** For example, by consuming milk products. If you have a lactose intolerance, eat lactose-poor cheese, like cheddar.

**Omega 3:** For example, by eating flaxseeds or their oil, rapeseed oil or fish.

Also, ensure to eat a variety of foods, to supply your body with the vitamins that are important for your health. To do so, regularly eat fruits and vegetables.

# 2.2 Your individual strategy

**T**his Chapter describes how to proceed accurately with the introduction of diet and the sensitivity level test. During the introductory diet, you keep the portions stated in the tables in Chapter 3. Please note here that the tolerated portions refer to one meal—expecting three meals at intervals of about six hours per day. Follow these steps to find out if the diet has an effect:

First, you take the introductory diet according to the food tables in Chapter 3. Four days before starting the diet as well as on the last four days of the third week, you fill out the symptom test sheet on page 27. With it, you can determine the diet's success, see chapter 4.3. The diet is efficient; however, if after three weeks of keeping it, you should not find any improvement, find out whether you unwillingly consumed too much lactose. One way to investigate this is to keep a nutrition diary and check it with a specialist or nutrition consultant. If you ruled out an accidental intake of lactose, and are unhappy with the improvement of your well-being, you may be more sensitive than is normal—try half the amounts in the lactose lists to find out. In addition, work on your stress level see Chapter 2.8. Aside from that, you can use *THE IBS NAVIGATOR* to test for a fructans and galactans sensitivity that often accompanies a lactose intolerance as well alternative trigger.

## The test procedure in three levels of escalation

Subsequently, you find an example of the test process:
1) Reduce your lactose consumption according to the lactose tables in Chapter 3 for three weeks. Fill out the symptom test sheet for four days before the diet as well as on the last four days. In the third week, if your discomforts improved satisfactory, keep the lactose diet. If you like, you can adjust your sensitivity level further (see Chapter 4). If you remain dissatisfied, act according to step 2).
2) Work on your stress management see Chapter 2.8.
3) Get *THE IBS NAVIGATOR* and repeat the introduction with fructans and galactans as well. Did your symptoms improve further? If so, keep this diet. In case you are still searching for an improvement, check the alternative strategies chapter in that book.

## 2.2.1 Substitute test

You want to check, whether you can stomach lactose but your expert is unable to offer you a breath test? For this case, I have developed the substitute test. As you determine the result based on your symptoms, it is necessary to rule out the influence of alternative triggers. Thus, you need *THE IBS NAVIGATOR* to do the test. In it, you will find the extensive explanation and the instruction to perform the substitute test.

## 2.2.2 It depends on the total load

You feel discomfort as soon as too much of lactose arrives at your small intestine for your enzyme workers to handle. The more lactose, the worse your symptoms are. In the food tables in the third part of the book, you will find the portion sizes that fit. What do you do if you want to combine different foods, e.g., as you prepare to cook a recipe, if you tolerate a limited amount of some of them? If you used the maximum amount of lactose on the milk for the rice pudding already, do you have to deny yourself the vanilla sauce? Nonessential: reduce the consumption for one or several of the affected foods far enough to not surpass the amount thresholds in sum. Makes sense? Not yet? Here is another example: you want to drink condensed milk in your coffee for breakfast (the tolerable amount is half a portion of 31 mL), and you love mascarpone as a spread (your acceptable portion size for it is 2¼ portions of 30g each). Hence, both foods contain lactose. In order not to surpass your tolerance threshold, restrict yourself to ¼ of a portion of condensed milk (about two teaspoons—10 mL) and one portion of mascarpone. Thus, the total amount of lactose you consume at the meal is below your threshold. If the reduced amounts are too small for you, you may want to look for alternatives. In Chapter 3.4.3, you can find various cold cut. Your tolerable portion size for Cheddar cheese, for example, is quite high.

# 2.3 Prevalence of the intolerances

According to an extensive current study in Switzerland, 27% of people with abdominal discomfort suffer from a fructose intolerance, 17% from a lactose intolerance and a further 33% from both. However, the fructose dose of 35g that the study used is high for European conditions, if a Finnish study from 1987 still applies to contemporary diets, and low for American conditions, wherein the average daily amount consumed is 54g. Hence, there is no fixed reference around the world. Another research study using 25g fructose as its base level suggests only a 49% average prevalence of fructose intolerance. An analysis of several studies shows that independent from the investigations mentioned above, 58% of those with irritable bowel symptoms have a sorbitol intolerance. There are no research results concerning the prevalence of a fructans and galactans intolerance known to me at this point.

Are you surprised about the low level of lactose intolerance? Well, you have to account for the fact that it is lowest for Caucasians as they adapted to tolerate milk to cope better with less sunshine in a day. Still, I was amazed that lactose intolerance is not the common type of intolerances according to the studies I read. If you stroll through supermarkets, however, you will hardly find a shelf that holds products for people with sorbitol or fructose intolerance. Instead, the markets have adjusted solely on lactose intolerance—also concerning the labeling. From this perspective, it is better to be lactose intolerant.

# 2.4   General diet hints

## 2.4.1   Good reasons for your persistence

I magine that one of your best friends goes on a two-week vacation leaving his beloved Labrador retriever, *Bailey*, in your care, along with some instructions about the dog's health needs as it has an intolerance towards an ingredient in some dog foods. You run out of dog food after the first week, just as you sat down on the couch to relax—not planning to leave the house again for today. Now you remember that you still have a can of the food you give to the square like dog of your auntie in the basement. If you give *Bailey* some of that, you save an hour drive to the store and back as well as going outside where it started to rain. Annoyingly, the food for your aunt's dog contains the trigger *Bailey* has to avoid. Unlike the happy dog image on the package suggests, giving him this food causes him pain, flatulence, and lethargy; catching a stick will be out of the question for this poor pooch. Maybe, you also imagine your aunt, whose dog feels well, even after consuming what you would never feed him— you remember a cream pie that fell victim to that bitch. "Hogwash!" she would say. "Dogs can eat anything! A dog intolerance? If he only eats enough there will be no farts!"

What is your position at that moment? Back on the couch or driving through the rain to the expert dealer? Now, I am relieved. Therefore, the dog of your friend is worth spending time and money as well as acting considerably. If, at any point it becomes difficult for you to keep your diet, think about the happy *Bailey* and send the square couch potato dog back to your aunt's home!

In the end, I call upon you to take responsibility for your nutrition. Show respect to your body. Acquire the necessary courage and discipline. Your body is a part of you. Just as many vegetarians stand by their dietary choices for the duration of their lives, you should stand by your diet and your body. Be yourself. The key is not starting out perfect, but starting at all and making small improvements every day. That is something you can do! You have the courage and *Bailey* will give you the courage.

Your target should be to change your sustenance day by day, food by food, in such a way as to allow you to lead a mostly symptom-free life. All beginnings are difficult, however, and as you leap the initial hurdles, you will find further motivation and discipline in discovering how much your nutritional changes are paying off for you.

The first step in that direction is to connect that goal with whatever is most important to you in your life. Independent of where your passions lie, you will enjoy them better by gaining more energy and improved wellbeing.

Do you not believe me? The retriever sneaks through the house and as he sees a cat pass by through the window, his only reaction is to fart, then, he retreats into his dog hatchet with an abdominal cramp. Curing the food for aunt's dog that got him into the hot water – you do not want to end up likewise. What about this instead: The retriever sneaks through the house, hears steps, stalks to the open window, stops and sees what looks like a burglar nearby the post box (he does not see the letters in his hands). In a flash, *Bailey* is on the road right behind him giving him a good bark! Pure energy!

What triggers your passion? What is your affair of the heart? Gain strength by keeping a diet that is best for you and give it a fresh start. Turn your attention and abilities toward eating in a way that will help you achieve your goals. If you are uncertain whether you can reach, your goals do this: Imagine that you have already done it. How? Cut out the following card and fold it as indicated. Then put it somewhere you can see it every day. Ideally, you can take a picture of yourself after a particularly fruitful milestone and put it on the drawing. Then let it encourage you to continue improving your nutrition each day. *Stephen William Hawking* has never stopped producing outstanding scientific works despite suffering from a myasthenia. Why? Because he is following his heart and because he has a positive attitude about life. Who seeks excuses when they are passionate about something? When it comes to passion, it is all about the how. It is about doing what is possible and thus it is always all about the solution. There are similar examples in sports. *Melissa Stockwell* achieves first class athletic performance despite having lost a leg. Her sport is her passion, and she finds ways to excel in it regardless of the circumstances life gave her.

So what is your passion? Write it down. Then make it clear to yourself that a symptom-reducing diet will positively affect your achievement. Then get on your way to making this nutrition a part of your life. In addition—always remember about your friend, *Bailey,* the dog.

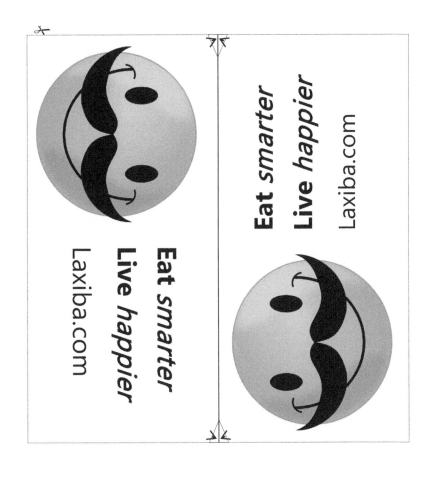

## 2.4.2  Mealtimes

Even when and how often you eat can affect your digestion. Who better to ask on that subject than athletes? They, in particular, depend on an optimal nutrient supply. The analysis shows that over 97% of elite Canadian athletes eat at least three times a day; 57% of them also take a snack in the morning, 71% in the afternoon and 58% in the evening. Moreover, regular mealtimes have a positive effect on the cardiovascular system. A study of more than 4,500 children showed that the risk of childhood obesity markedly decreases the more often children eat during the day. How is that? Well, ask the mail carrier of *Bailey's* owner, whether he dares bringing him his letters after eating a gravitationally detrimental meal, his daily ration, in the morning.

## 2.4.3  Eating out

At home, restricting one's consumption of lactose containing foods is rather easy. Now you want to eat at a restaurant of a friend's house so what do you do? Of course, you understand that a restaurant staff usually does not have the dietician's expertise required to tell you the ingredients of each meal. Luckily, you can help yourself. For example by learning about some foods that you can usually eat without having to think about them. These include eggs, fish or meat without breading or sauce, kiwis, leafy salads dressed with oil, oregano, pepper and salt, oranges, basil pesto, potatoes, rice, and tortillas. What about menus, however? Have you ever spent time at a restaurant considering what the ideal combination of menu items would be for you? The good thing is that you can often ask for a change to menu items without paying extra if you ask the server. You can likewise voice your needs to your hosts when you receive an invitation to a meal. To make it easy, just hand out the safe products list (see Chapter 2.6). You can send it out with the following message, for example:

*"Dear [name of the host],*

*I was glad to receive your invitation to [occasion like your wedding], and I am happy to come. If it is possible for you to cook some of the foods that are included in the attached table separately from the other meals, then I can take part in the meal, as well. Please tell me whether that will be possible so that I can plan accordingly.*

*Thank you and see you soon!*

*[Your name]"*

The safe products list, see Chapter 2.6, also makes it easier for a restaurant kitchen to find a suitable meal for you. As fast food chains are not as readily equipped to adapt their menus, you will find many fast food chain products and the portion sizes you can stomach in the third part of this book. You can stay on the safe side by always having your book with you. However, it will hardly be always at hand, unlike a foldable list for your purse or wallet. In Chapter 2.5 you will find the cheat sheet with the tolerable portion sizes of some common products.

## 2.4.4  Convenience foods

Unfortunately, lactose is a part of many convenience foods or are naturally contained in the ingredients. However, you will find exceptions, even when shopping on the cheap, including convenience foods that advertise the use of natural ingredients—check the ingredient list.

## 2.4.5  Medicine and oral hygiene

Anything you take into your mouth can cause symptoms if it contains lactose. When considering medicines that include lactose, take into account the amount you can stomach at your sensitivity level, which is 3g for the standard level. It helps to know that middle-sized capsules contain 0.58g at the most, and the largest, 1.6g per piece while tablets are usually even a little lighter. For mixtures, a teaspoon holds about 5 ml/g and a tablespoon 5–15 ml/g.

Despite your best efforts at researching your intolerance, you may find yourself unable to stomach medicine for whatever reason. If you are having symptoms, search for alternatives. If in doubt, use the symptom-test-sheet. Write down your symptoms while using it and compare it with a record of your diet taken when you were not using the medicine, for example, on your efficiency check sheet. You can use any sheet where you recorded your symptoms after refraining from lactose.

## 2.4.6    Nutritional supplements

If you take vitamin supplements, the following examples are lactose-free:

*Nature's Bounty® Vitamin B-12*, 1000mcg, *Nature Made® Vitamin B6 100mg* Dietary Supplement Tablets, *Walgreens® Multivitamin Ultimate Men's Tablets*, *Walgreens® Multivitamin Ultimate Women's Tablets*. A long-term trial did not prove the use of multivitamin supplements. If you take them, make sure not to take too much of certain vitamins. Vitamins that can be unsafe in excess include *B3, B6*, as well as *A, D, E* and *K*, which can cause symptoms of poisoning if you overdose. Thus, you should discuss your intake with your doctor. A viable approach with these vitamins is taking them in three-month cycles. That means taking them for three months and then taking the next three months off.

## 2.4.7    Fish and meat

Fish and meat by nature are free of lactose. Nevertheless, you have to be careful with breaded fish and meat, processed such as bratwurst or liverwurst and sauce—these may contain lactose. To find out about included that, check the list of ingredients of the product.

## 2.4.8    These actions lead to lasting change

To achieve lasting success, it is important that you monitor your nutrition. If you find yourself starting to ignore the recommended amounts, you should get back on track and restart your commitment as soon as possible. Write down your goal to adapt your nutrition to the stated food and drink portion sizes to reduce abdominal discomfort and improve your quality of life. Stay conscious of the negative consequences of eating "blindly" covered in the first part of this book. Why is it important to change your habits? Re-read your goal and then write down your five most important reasons for striving toward it. Moreover, answer the following question. Why it is important to act **now**?

Probably, you have made the following experience as well. Filled with motivation and enthusiasm you plunge into something, like a New Year's resolution. One goes right after it and even celebrates first successes. However, this feeling trickles away unless soon afterward even bigger successes surpass the first one. If that does not happen, a slight inertia arises. If you change your diet, this can happen to you as well. It is like there is an angel on your one shoulder to whom you say that you are going to keep at it even if it becomes arduous yet there is an imp sitting on your other shoulder, which is already laughing at his sleeve. In fact, the way gets steeper after the first yards. Many then let things slide, which makes further successes impossible, and the symptoms come back. "Isn't that unfair?" the imp is telling you, "you are putting in your effort for days and how does it pay off? You are having the same symptoms as you had before. Let it be." The angel may have screamed so much that it is croaky by now and shrugs his shoulders exhaustedly. "Sorry, but I tried my best," one excuses oneself trying not to look at the grinning devil.

It is a cognitive bias to believe that it is easier just to accept one's symptoms than to change your diet to avoid them. What about you? Did you catch yourself close to giving up? If so, send the devil on your shoulder to the desert where it belongs.

I can promise you: After you changed your diet to fit your food's lactose content, you will have more energy and a higher quality of life. In addition, after you have mastered staying on the right path for some month, you will find that you are getting used to it, which will make it even easier to stick with it. Getting used to it is something that the imp has deliberately concealed: Once you have taken the first pitch, you get accustomed to quickly assessing foods about their content of the lactose and learns to notice lactose hideouts. Juggling with the amounts becomes so easy that you do not have to think long. At the start, the cheat sheet and this book will serve you well. Later you no longer need both as you know yourself what is right for you. The imp that you sent to the desert now is hot with anger, and you are the one that has a big grin on the face. You have the best arguments to be tenacious!

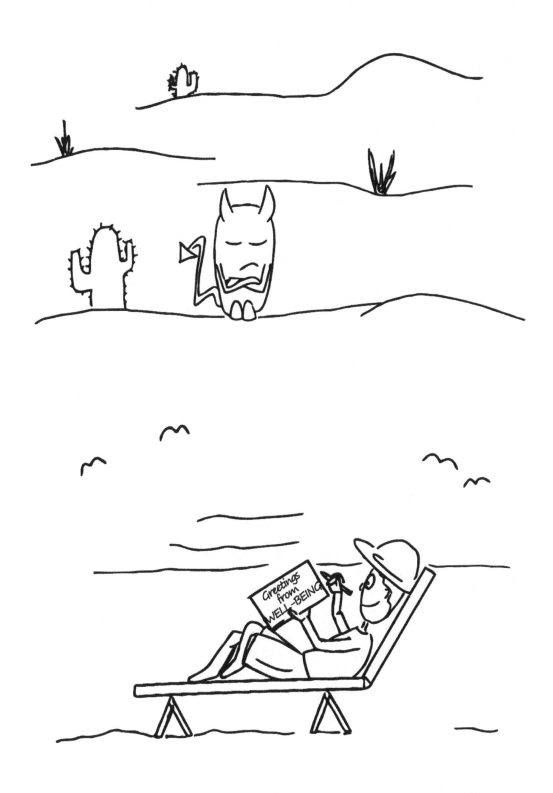

Are you uncertain as to whether you are going to remain motivated? Create an objective agreement with yourself. Note down in writing, why it pays off to you, to endure. Which goal do you want to achieve? For example, like this:

## Objective agreement (write it down yourself)

**What:** comply with the acceptable amounts – Send the devil to the desert.

**How to measure it:** daily at 7:45 pm (set an alarm on your phone): did I eat dairy products and comply with the portion restrictions?

**Consequence:** YES, you complied, so give yourself a small reward. NO, you did not so do 10 pushups or mow the lawn (anything you can do, which is good for you but you do not like doing).

**Get it done:** start within three days and keep on actively managing your diet until you have formed a habit of doing it.

**Activities:** Put this book into your kitchen and the cheat sheet into your wallet; inform those close to you; create reminders in your flat and your car, place your objective agreement somewhere where you can see it at least once a day (e.g. your mirror).

A good way to ensure that you stay committed is to integrate your spouse. Ask them to motivate you and to reflect back to you, which positive changes they notice about you. Another option is to book one of our coaches at *https://laxiba.com/trainer* to help you implement the steps explained in this book. What is more, you will find a way to talk with others and motivate each other at *https://laxiba.com/team*.

The more vivid and multifaceted you can imagine your life after a successful conversion of your diet, the more likely you are to keep moving forward with it and doing what is necessary. Have you been in a rut one day? Forget about it; get the job done better the day after! You can use this book as a compass and correct your course back to being well!

## 2.4.9   Reasons for using the triggers

Why for example is lactose contained in some drugs or sausages? These products have nothing to do with milk! There is a swift explanation. When it comes to processed food, lactose creates certain flavors, makes sausages thicker and saves money. For drugs, lactose is a carrier for active substances because it is simple and works well. There would be alternatives that work well in many cases, which would not cost much more. So far, there is no strong lobby against using lactose in foods or making them easier to avoid, yet. Of course, lactose also occurs naturally, but that is not a valid reason to use it in, for example, medicine.

## 2.4.10  Positive aspects of the diet

Do you want to disagree with me after reading the headline? For many the lactose diet equals abdication. In its original sense, however, diet (from the Greek díaita) means "lifestyle" or "way of life." Are abdication and the feeling of a downer an accurate description of the lifestyle that you want? On the contrary, you perform the diet to lower you symptoms and thus increases your quality of life. As you find out, which foods you can eat concerning their lactose content, you will automatically start thinking about what you eat in general. The chances are that you will end up eating healthier, and healthy is a much friendlier summary of your lifestyle. Of course, an alternative to the diet would be the use of medicine, like painkillers or drugs to stop diarrhea. Better yet, is to make sure symptoms do not occur in first place. You can also use lactase enzymes, which also achieves the latter aim, although as you will learn the food lists for many dairy products, the tolerated amount is larger than you might guess.

## 2.4.11  Testing yourself

Some of those affected by lactose intolerace reportedly struggle to absorb other ingredients like aspartame or maltodextrin. Apart from that, a sensitivity towards fructans and galactans is common. So if your symptoms prevail, check fructans and galactans as well as an alternative introductory diet outlined in *THE IBS NAVIGATOR*.

# Summary

A healthy, balanced diet, fixed mealtimes, and regular exercise are important not only in case of a lactose intolerance but for all people. Unfortunately, sometimes lactose is included in products although lactose free alternatives are available. Hence, especially when eating convenience foods or taking drugs, watch out for lactose in the ingredients. Stick to the lactose diet if it works. The longer you persist, the easier it gets to maintain it.

# 2.5   The cheat sheet

Cut out the leaflet on the following page. Please fold it along the thick lines. Start with the dotted line. Then fold it again at the half-dashed line. You can now keep this important information at hand when you are out and about or shopping.

## Cheat sheet content

Here you can find information on lactose-containing foods. Asian, Greek, Italian and Spanish meals usually contain little lactose. Fish, other seafood, meat, black coffee, eggs, and oils are also free from lactose. The same holds for fruits and vegetable.

| Despite their name, these ingredients are free from lactose | | |
| --- | --- | --- |
| Milk acid | Glucono delta-lactone | Rice and almond milk |
| Milk protein | Lactose freed milk products | |
| Lactate, lactase | INS additive numbers: 575, 325-327 | |

| These products contain lactose | | |
| --- | --- | --- |
| Lactose | Yogurt | Whey |
| Cheese | Kefir, lassi | Milk(-powder) |
| Curd | (Concentrated) butter | Cream |

## Attention, lactose is often contained in:

- Cereals
- Ice cream and sweets like chocolate
- Coffee and milk, condensed milk
- Dairy products, like milk, curd, and yogurt
- Breading, sauces, puréed meat, tzatziki
- Sweet pastries like biscuits, cakes, and tarts, cream

Front **Flyer for lactose intolerance**

### Free of lactose despite their name are:

| | | |
|---|---|---|
| Milk acid | Glucono delta- | Rice and |
| Milk protein | lactone | almond milk |
| Lactate | Lactose freed milk products | |
| Lactase | (INS additive numbers: 575, 325-327) | |

### Products containing lactose:

| | | |
|---|---|---|
| Lactose | Whey | Yoghurt |
| Cheese | Kefir, lassi | Milk(-powder) |
| Curd | Cream | (Concentrated) butter |

Asian, Greek, Italian and Spanish meals contain little lactose. Asian rice meals also containing few fructans and galactans. Fish, seafood, meat, black coffee, eggs and oils are also free from lactose. The same holds for fruits and vegetable although some of them contain fructans and galactans.

Back **More lactose sources:** LAXIBA®

- Cereals
- Ice cream and sweets like chocolate
- Coffee and milk, condensed milk
- Dairy products, like cream, curd and yoghurt
- Breading, sauces, puréed meat, Tzatziki
- Sweet pastries—biscuits, cakes, tarts, & cream

## Interior left **Lactose intolerance:**

| | |
|---|---|
| Apple | Oranges |
| Apricot | Parmesan |
| Carrots | Pear |
| celery | Peppers |
| Chocolate sorbet | Potatoes |
| Coconut | Rice |
| Drinks without | Spelt flour |
| milk, yoghurt, etc. | Squash |

Fish and Meat Jelly babies Ice tea Ketchup Kiwi Lettuce Oil & vinegar

## Low lactose content for average serving sizes

Butter☺; 14g  Margarine²¹³⁄₄P.; 9g  Swiss
Cheddar³³¼P.; 30g  Nutella®³²¾P.; 37g  cheese
Fondue sauce☺; 53g  Parmesan☺; 5g  ☺; 30g

Per active lactase capsule you take in, you can stomach about 75% more of each shown serving size.

### These are the portion unit abbreviations:

| Exemplar | Cup | Glas | Portion | Slice |
|---|---|---|---|---|
| E | C | G | P | S |

☹=avoid; ☺=nearly free; ☺☺=is free of it

## Interior right **Products with a high amount of lactose**

| | | |
|---|---|---|
| Cacao¼C.; 150g | Kefir¼P.; 220g | Mozzarella9¾P.30g |
| Casserole½P.; 238g | Mashed- | Pancake½P.; 187g |
| Cheese-sauce¼P.; 66g | potatoe¼P.; 140g | Tart½P.; 87,5g |
| Condensed milk½P | Milk rice¼P.; 107g | Yoghurt¼P.; 250g |
| Creme-soup½P.; 245g | Milk¼C.; 200g | |

# 2.6   The safe products list

Likely, kely, if you yourself do not have a lactose intolerance, someone in your circle of acquaintances has the irritable bowel syndrome or an intolerance towards some ingredient. As a good host, you may have already been in a situation to consider those to make sure that none of your guests encounters an uneasy feeling after an invitation.

If you ask your guests to tell you about any problematic ingredient you should accustom to, you are prepared professionally: Such a question will always leave a positive impression as it shows that your guest's well-being is important to you. You are well accustomed to any guest, if you make sure that some foods that are usually tolerable for anyone are on the menu. How can you achieve that? It is quite simple: make sure to offer the sauces separately from the side dishes. Hence, provide a bowl of potatoes, another bowl with butter, a third one with salad and lastly one with dressings. By the way, with some exceptions like garlic and onions anyone can tolerate most herbs and spices. The table on the following page shows you some usually safe foods.

| Fruit | Vegetables | Warm dishes |
|---|---|---|
| Blackberries | Avocado, green | Brandy vinegar |
| Currants | Basil | Caviar |
| Dates, fresh | Chard | Chinese oyster sauce |
| Figs, fresh | Chives | Fish, meat, shrimp and |
| Goji berries | Coriander | shellfish* |
| Lemon zest | Green peppers | Kraft® Italian Dressing |
| Loganberry | Horseradish | |
| Papaya | Kelp | Kraft® Mayonnaise |
| Passion fruit | Oregano | Oils |
| Rhubarb | Parsnips | Kraft® Thousand Island |
| | Peppermint, fresh | Dressing® |
| | Rice | Pepper and salt |
| | Rosemary | Rice bread |
| | Rutabaga | Rice noodles |
| | Squash: Butternut, calabash, giant and spaghetti | Soy oil |
| | Thyme | Spelt flour |
| | Yam | Tabasco® sauce |

*Non pureed and without breading and sauce.

| Beverages | | Other |
|---|---|---|
| Black coffee | Baking powder | Pecan nuts |
| Brandy | Brazil nuts | Pine nuts |
| Gin | Brown sugar | Pistachios |
| Jasmine tea | Cashews | Pumpkin seeds |
| Maté tea | Coconut | Rice bread |
| Peppermint tea | Gelatin | Spelt |
| Rum | Ginkgo | Walnuts |
| Tequila | Licorice | White sugar |
| Tonic Water | Macadamia nuts | |
| Vodka | Maple syrup | |
| Water | Peanut butter | |
| Whiskey | Peanuts | |

# 2.7 Recipes

## 2.7.1 Apricot cuts

**Tolerable amount concerning the lactose content: as much as you like**

**What you need:**

4 tbsp. of apricot jam
4/5 cup of dried, fine sliced apricots
One cup of butter
One cup of flour (in case of celiac disease, use gluten free flour)
3/5 cup of rice flour
One tsp. of vanilla-extract
2/5 cup of sugar, as well as some to dust over

**Preparation:**

Preheat the oven at 390 °F top and bottom heat or 360 °F convection heat. Then, lay out an eight in deep backing tray with baking paper. Now add the apricots and jam in a small pan with 4 tbsp. water. Simmer over medium heat until they are thick. Then squash the apricots a little with a fork and let them cool down. Add the butter, vanilla extract and sugar in a bowl and mix with the blender. Afterward, add the rice flour and the flour and whip with a spoon or your hands to form a dough. Then, divide the dough into two equal pieces. Spread one-half of the dough on the baking sheet. Knead the remaining dough into an eight in² square piece and place it on top. Press alongside the edge of the dough and stab some small holes into it with a fork. Bake for 25-30 minutes until the corners turn golden. Leave it in the baking mold for the cool down and sprinkle powdered sugar over it. Slice three cuts to the top and the sides and that is it.

## 2.7.2   Banana cake

**Tolerable amount concerning the lactose content: as much as you like**

**What you need:**

Two ripe bananas
A handful of banana chips
One packet of baking powder (celiac disease? Use gluten-free baking powder)
3/5 cup of butter and something for the baking mold
Two large eggs
1/5 cup of icing
3/5 cup of flour (use gluten free flour if gluten intolerant)
3/5 cup of sugar

**Preparation:**

Preheat the oven to 390 °F top and bottom heat or 360 °F circulating air. Meanwhile spread some butter into a marble cake mold. Gently mix the butter and sugar together. Then slowly add the eggs and some flour. Afterward, stir the rest of the flour, baking powder and bananas into the mix. Place the dough in a baking mold and bake the cake for about 30 minutes until it well rises. Now let it cool down in the mold for about 10 minutes. Following, prepare the frosting with two teaspoons of water, douse the cake with it and decorate with the banana chips.

## 2.7.3　Creamy rice pudding

**Tolerable amount concerning the lactose content: as much as you like**

**What you need** (for four servings):

One tbsp. butter

2/5 cup of cranberries

One egg

3/5 cup of rice

2 cups of rice milk

One pinch of salt

½ tsp. of vanilla extract

¼ cup of sugar

**Preparation:**

Cook the rice in water. Then add 350g of cooked rice with ¾ of the milk, the sugar and a pinch of salt in a new pan, stir from time to time and let the mix cook for another 3 minutes. Meanwhile, beat the egg in a small bowl with a wire whisk. At the end of the cooking time, add to the mix with the rest of the milk and the cranberries and let it simmer it yet another 3 minutes. It is important that you always stir it. Now remove the pan from the plate and mix with the butter and the vanilla extract - Bon appetite.

## 2.7.4 Fruit salad

**Tolerable amount concerning the lactose content: as much as you like**

**What you need** (four servings):

4/5 cup of pineapple
One banana, ½ cup
One cup of strawberry
One orange, 3/5 cup
One cup of cranberries
One tbsp. of lemon juice

**Preparation:**

Peel the pineapple, remove the stem and cut into finger-thick pieces. Now peel the orange, remove the seeds and chop up, also cut the strawberries. Place the pieces in a bowl and pour the lemon juice over them. Stir well now and you did it.

# 2.7.5   Fruit salad with curd

**Tolerable amount concerning the lactose content: 3 and ¼ servings**

**What you need** (eight servings):

Maple syrup
Two cups of canned pineapple (if fresh the curd turns bitter)
One and ¼ cup of cranberries
One and ¼ cup of canned mandarins
Two cups of sour cream or cottage cheese with a little milk

**Preparation:**

Cut the pineapple into finger-thick pieces. Now place the fruit and sour cream in a bowl. After stirred well, season well with the maple syrup. To consume enough glucose-containing cranberries, puree the fruits with a blender.

## 2.7.6 Lemon bar

**Tolerable amount concerning the lactose content: 10 pieces**

**What you need:**
**For the dough:**

3/5 cup of butter
¾ cup of flour (celiac disease? Use gluten free flour)
One tbsp. milk
1/5 cup of rice flour
4/5 cup of brown sugar

**For the topping:**

Three eggs
2 tbsp. of flour (celiac disease? Use gluten free flour)
Icing sugar
The zest of three lemons
4/5 cup of mL lemon juice
4/5 cup of sugar

**Preparation:**

Preheat the oven at 430 °F top and bottom heat or 390 °F air circulation. Cover a 9 in. baking tray with baking paper. Mix the butter, the flour, rice flour and sugar in a bowl, until only small lumps form. Then add the milk and spread the dough on the baking tray. Let it bake for 17 minutes until golden brown. Then remove the tray and reduce the oven temperature to 390 °F top and bottom heat or 360 °F air circulation. Whisk the lemon juice and the eggs, the sugar, the flour and the lemon zest in a bowl. Pour this concentrate over the dough and bake the lemon bars for another 15 minutes until the surface almost firm. Let it cool down on the tray. Finally, cut and powder - ready to enjoy.

## 2.7.7 Pancakes

**Tolerable amount concerning the lactose content: as much as you like**

**What you need:**

One egg
Half a cup of flour (celiac disease? Use gluten free flour)
1 and ¼ cup of rice milk
Sunflower oil

**Preparation:**

Put the flour into a bowl and make a hole in the middle, in which you put the egg together with the rice milk. Now whisk everything well with a mixer. Add a quarter of the rice milk and continue to add the rest once the batter is lump free. Now let the dough rest and after 20 minutes whisk it again. Preheat a small non-stick frying pan and pour the oil into it. Cover the whole bottom of the pan with a thin layer of dough. Fry the pancakes on each side, until golden brown. Place some baking paper between the pancakes when you pile them, so they remain crispy. Serve with any filling.

## 2.7.8  Pizza dough

**Tolerable amount concerning the lactose content: as much as you like**

**What you need:**

7g (one filled tsp) yeast (celiac disease? Use dry gluten-free yeast. First, let it rise with a tsp. of sugar in a cup that is half-full of water. After that, mix it with the rest of the water and flour. Often, it takes some time until the dough has risen.)
One and ½ cups of flour (celiac disease? Use gluten-free flour, here you may have to experiment a bit)
One 1/5 cups of water

**Preparation:**

Put the flour with a tsp. salt, yeast and 275 mL lukewarm water in a bowl and mix everything for about 5 minutes to form a dough. Now, take out the dough and let it rise it in a lightly oiled bowl until it rises about twice the size. Knead the dough afterwards for a bit, then cut it in half and roll out each of both parts on a thin layer of flour as thin as possible. Now garnish the pizza as desired and bake in the oven at 430 °F air circulation.

# 2.7.9   Rhubarb, roasted

**Tolerable amount concerning the lactose content: as much as you like**

**What you need** (five servings):

1 and 1/3 cup of Rhubarb
1/3 cup of brown sugar

**Preparation:**

Preheat the oven at 390 °F top and bottom heat or 360 °F air circulation. Wash the Rhubarb then shake off the water. Cut the end and the middle of the sticks into small finger-sized pieces. Cover a closed baking tray with a baking sheet and spread the Rhubarb on it. Sprinkle some sugar over it and cover the Rhubarb with it. Bake the Rhubarb for about 15 minutes with baking paper on top. Then remove the baking paper and shake the plate slightly. Then continue baking for about five minutes. When the Rhubarb is ready, it is soft, but not mushy.

# 2.7.10 Rhubarb cake

**Tolerable amount concerning the lactose content: as much as you like**

**What you need:**

One packet of baking powder (celiac disease? Use gluten-free baking powder)
Four large eggs
One cup of flour (celiac disease? Use gluten free flour)
Icing sugar
Pre-roasted Rhubarb, as described before.
One cup of sweet cream butter and even something for the baking tray
One tsp. vanilla extract
3/5 cup of custard
One cup of brown sugar

**Preparation:**

First, prepare the roasted Rhubarb and drain the juice. Preheat now the oven at 390 °F top and bottom heat or 180 degrees air circulation. Wipe a nine in cake springform pan with butter. Put 3 tbsp. of the vanilla pudding in a separate bowl. The rest you whisk up creamy with butter, the flour, baking powder, eggs and sugar in a bowl. Pour one-third of the mix in the cake form and place about half of the Rhubarb over it. Put one more third of dough over this layer and flatten it as smooth as possible. Cover the top with the rest of the Rhubarb and pour the remaining mixture over it, this time, the surface remains rough. Then use the remaining 3 tbsp. of the vanilla pudding to place on top. Bake the cake for 40 minutes, until it rises and becomes golden. Cover it with baking paper and leave it baking for another 15 minutes. The cake is ready when you stab it with a toothpick, and it comes out clean. Sprinkle some icing sugar over the cake after it cooled down.

# 2.7.11 Rhubarb-smoothie

**Tolerable amount concerning the lactose content: as much as you like**

**What you need** (for two servings):

One small banana
One cup of cranberry juice
2/5 cup of frozen Rhubarb
Five tbsp. (1/2 cups) of vanilla yogurt or lactose-free vanilla yogurt (1/2 cup)

**Preparation:**

Cut the banana into small pieces and puree everything together in a blender.

# 2.7.12 Rucola salad

**Tolerable amount concerning the lactose content: ½ serving**

**What you need** (for 2-3 servings):

Four tsp. vinegar from vinegar essence-water mixture
Two cups of grill cheese (e.g., halumi)
Three tbsp. of olive oil
Three medium, skinned oranges
One small bunch of chopped peppermint
3/5 cup of Rocket salad
1/5 cup (3 tbsp.) of roasted walnuts

**Preparation:**

Heat up a pan in which you fry the 1/3 in. sized grill cheese slices for about 1 to 2 minutes until they begin to melt. Mix the oranges with the juice from the peeling; the mint leaves and the vinegar gently in a bowl. Now add the walnuts and the rocket salad and mix well. Place the cheese slices on top. Finally, season the salad with black pepper - good appetite.

# 2.7.13 Spaghetti al salmone

**Tolerable amount concerning the lactose content: 10 pieces**

**What you need** (for 2-3 portions):

Two small finely ground chillies
Four tbsp. capers without the water from the glass
Two cloves of garlic
½ cup of mL extra virgin olive oil
4/5 cup of rocket salad
Two cups of spaghetti (celiac disease? Use gluten-free pasta)
200g salmon pieces
Two tbsp. of small cubes of white bread (celiac disease? Use gluten-free bread
or go without croutons)
Lemon zest, meaning the yellow skin of a well-washed lemon

**Preparation:**

Heat up two tbsp. of olive oil in the pan and toast in the bread cubes over medium heat for three to four minutes, until golden brown. Place in a small bowl afterwards. Cook the spaghetti in salted water until al dente. Meanwhile, squeeze out the garlic cloves and heat the garlic with the chili powder and the remaining oil in the pan. Please make sure not to fry the garlic. Let the pasta drain and place them in a preheated bowl. Next, put the grated lemon zest and capers into the oil. Pour it over the pasta and spread it well. At last, you mix everything with the salmon and the rocket salad. Sprinkle the croutons over it before serving—et voila.

# 2.7.14 Sweet potato- or salami & pesto-pizza

**Tolerable amount concerning the lactose content: ¼ of one pizza**

**What you need** (for two servings):

3/5 cup of ciabatta bread-dough mixture
½ cup of mozzarella balls
Two tsp. Olive oil, one for pizza and one for the baking tray
Two tbsp. green pesto
A handful of rocket salad
4/g cup of sweet potatoes (or salami)

**Preparation:**

Peel the potatoes, cut them into slices and boil them for 15 minutes in salted water. Then drain and let cool down briefly. Meanwhile, preheat the oven to 430 °F. Form the dough into a pizza shape and place it on a pre-oiled baking sheet. Now wait for 15 minutes. Spread the pesto on the pizza base. Sprinkle half of the mozzarella over it. The next layer is the potatoes (or salami) and on top of it is the rest of the mozzarella. Let the pizza bake for 15 to 18 minutes until the crust is golden brown and the cheese bubbles. Finally, put the rocket salad on the pizza and season with black pepper.

# 2.7.15  Tuna pizza

**Tolerable amount concerning the lactose content: ¼ of one serving**

**What you need** (for eight servings):

A pack of cream cheese (225g)
2/3 cup of finely sliced mozzarella
Pepper
One and 2/3 cups (400g) pizza dough (celiac disease? Use gluten-free dough)
Small bunch chives
A can of tuna

**Preparation:**

Preheat the oven to 430 °F. Bake the dough briefly. Spread the cream cheese over it. Now cover the pizza base with tuna and mozzarella, season the pizza with pepper and finish baking. Meanwhile, wash the chives and cut it finely to spread it on the pizza, when it is ready.

# 2.8   Stress management

Stress can affect your stomach and worsen lactose intolerance symptoms. Hence, it is important to reduce it. To find out its effect on you, fill out your symptom-test-sheet on a day when you have a lot of stress. Developing a solution-oriented way to manage your worries can help you do so. How does that help? The more you stress over something, the more brain areas that you need for a reasonable decision are being set off. The body does so, because, in a certain way, our bodies are prepared for an earlier historical era. Dangerous situations like an attack by a wolf pack left us with three options: fight, flight or playing dead. If we spent too much time thinking in such a situation, it was game over! Hence, we are poled to stop thinking as soon as we feel we are in danger—which is not always helpful in our modern time.

If nowadays your boss storms into your office with some tricky and pressing demands of a huge client, neither a spontaneous attack nor jumping out of the window or acting as dead will be recommendable. Seriously, nowadays usually much different factors trigger stress than it was a few thousand years ago. Aside from noise, extreme temperatures, and air pollution, it is especially the feeling of losing control in a situation, which feels threatening to us. Fear can grab you, when a project is particularly delicate and important, something fundamental has to change, and you are under time pressure.

At the advent of fear, the release of hormones supports fight and flight reactions that enable us to make quick, even if ill-conceived, decisions. Everything inside of you screams "Do something immidiately, no matter what!" Large parts of our brain are set aside for that purpose. You feel stress and tend to make impulsive rather than rational decisions. The hormones lead to a shut down of vast areas of your brain at that moment; you feel stress. The third option your mind conceives in a dangerous situation, playing dead, somewhat corresponds to the extreme modern-day phenomena that is widely known as burnout.

So you have the impulses of a Stone Age hunter but the tasks of a top manager: how can you make that fit together? The only option you have to resist your impulse is to take command of your body and mind. To react appropriately, you are required not to have your hormones to turn off your resources for rational decision-making.

Once your body feels in danger, it is a challenge to halt the rolling wheel of your body's emergency reactions abruptly. Hence, the best thing you can do is to prevent these stress reactions from evolving in the first place. Yoga and progressive muscle relaxation before work are useful stress preventers. Using such techniques before going to work is sensible, as it is seldom possible to take an hour off during the workday. Breaks and disruptions during your working hours are also **counterproductive** if you are dealing with complex tasks; they often lead to poor decisions, more stress, and a short temper. Thus, try to avoid disruption when dealing with sophisticated tasks. You will agree if you imagine working on a complex calculation while your phone is ringing and your colleague enters to chat with you and a technician wanting to maintain your printer is waiting in front of the door. Therefore, try to avoid distractions when you are dealing with challenging tasks.

However, interruptions of simple mental or physical labor lasting a few minutes, rather than seconds, result in slight positive effects. Taking breaks from hard physical labor, meanwhile, show even stronger benefits, lowering the risk of injuries and enhancing endurance. You do not want to be following a printer printing during your break. To make the best use of it, close your eyes and focus on your breathing. Whenever thoughts come up, focus your whole attention bad on your breath without evaluating the thoughts. What makes this better is counting the times that you breathe out and feeling your breath leave your mouth.

Still, relaxation alone might not be the solution. Often, you can identify general worries that effect your mood. So how do you deal with such concerns? Many try to evade them by trying to ignore them, distract themselves or even take alcohol or other supposed comforters. Instead of bringing you closer to your goal, such a reaction, makes matters worse in most cases. The only thing that will help you resolve your troublesome thoughts is actively dealing with them. Only if you can name them, you can find solutions. Also, consider this; ignorance may well be one of the leading causes of failure.

Of course, for most worries no one hands you the solution on a silver platter. You have to take action. An open examination of your concerns and the right strategy can lead you towards a feasible solution. There is an immediate positive effect of this, independent from what solution you find: you avoid panic actions that one tends to in charged situations. If you regularly call a spade a spade and rationally seek solutions to situations you worry about you reduce the number of poor decisions.

By doing so, you can even use your fears—through the process of conquering them—to help you become more successful in your everyday life. What I recommend you do is sit down at a quiet desk at the beginning or end of the day. Next, think about what you are worried about right now and which steps you need to take to prevent the feared outcomes.

It is helpful to create an Excel spreadsheet for doing so or to purchase the standardized and printer-optimized edition at *www.Laxiba.com*. If you want to create the table by yourself, call the first sheet "Worries" and the second one "Task List." Next, write down the following task headings in the first spreadsheet: "Current Worries," "Preventive Measure A," "Preventive Measure B" and "Preventive Measure C." Then enter the following column titles in the second spreadsheet: "Task," "Priority," "Deadline," "Who does it?" and "Done."

You should write down your concerns in the first column of the first sheet. Then, think about what you will need to do to prevent these worries from becoming a reality. Think of three alternatives for each outcome. Enter these into the "Preventive Measure A–C" fields next to each worry, A being the action you want to take first. Then, transfer "Preventive Measure A" to the "Task List" sheet. Next, prioritize the tasks by employing an adapted version of the "Eisenhower method," an organization technique that takes importance and urgency into account, from A to E:

| Task is important | **A** *ction now* | **B** *etter do it soon* |
|---|---|---|
| Task is unimportant | **C** *hance to do the task if you completed all A and B duties.* | **D** *ull moment task* |
| **E** *fface, don't do task* | Task is urgent | Postponable task |

In the order from A to D, you then execute your duties on a daily basis. The category E is for tasks that are ineffective and therefore, you leave it. Hence, you prevent worrying and free yourself from doubting whether you are currently doing the right thing. After assessing the tasks from A to D, you fill out the column "Deadline," into which you enter the date at which you want to accomplish the task. Furthermore, you either note "I" or the name of the person that you want to delegate the work to in the column "Who does it?" Finally, you tick off the cell in the column „Done", when you have finished the task.

Another important aspect is keeping your life balanced. A fulfilled family life and friendships also help to improve your stress resistance. To name an example: taking a healthy exercise is beneficial for all areas of your life. Brought to an extreme, though, let's say if you spend ten hours per day at a fitness center, this will take too much of your time away from your other areas—unless you are a personal trainer. The four quadrants of your life are like the four legs of a stool you sit on. Let us call it your life-stool. If each leg is just as long as the others and all are adequately thick, you will sit well and safe. In however you chop off some from one or more legs repeatedly and strengthen another leg, you will start to waggle—until at some point, there is a crack, and you land on your patoot. You have to avoid this "breakdown". Of course, I know that this is exactly the dilemma that burdens many people nowadays. You feel that you have to perform continuously in all areas. Fathers do not only have to work. They also have to spend time with their family. They ought to bring their children to the violin tuition. Then in the evening, they should foster their social contacts and engage in the summer festival of their city. Having a well-trained body is necessary for many. On top of that, you ideally are relaxed and well groomed. For woman and mothers, the expectations are just as high. They feel like they have to perform like men at work and still manage their family, organize the spare time and stay fit. Expectations appear to rise everywhere.

So do not get me wrong: keeping your life in a healthy balance means finding the **right** balance between those things that are important to you personally. It is not about which expectations others have concerning your life's quadrants! It is not about what the society expects from you. What is important is that you consider the key aspects of your individual life. In the table below these are work, relaxation, family and spare time. For you, the quadrants may be different. You set the priorities yourself. Free yourself as much as possible from the influence of the acknowledgment by others, follow the saying "great horses jump tight" and develop a healthy self-confidence and composure.

Instead of delivering an over-the-top performance in one area but lousy results in all others, you want to do at least a satisfying job in all sectors, to remain capable in the end. Which of the family, spare time, relaxation and work quadrants are important is up to you, along with the results you are aiming for with them, such as spending time with those closest to you, taking daily walks, pursuing your hobbies and getting your work done properly. Furthermore, it is important to resist basing your success on external measures. You should nourish a healthy self-confidence and serenity in yourself. Thus, you need to know when finished the task you are doing well enough. Some people get into time trouble because they over deliver on some tasks and then have little time left to take care of other important tasks, which then causes stress. Often it takes 80% of the time to improve on the last 20% of a job, so it pays off if you know if the last 20% are worth it.

| **Family:** | **Relaxation:** |
|---|---|
| *Spend time with those closest to you* | *Go out for a walk on a daily basis* |
| **Spare time:** | **Work:** |
| *Pursue your hobbies regularly* | *Get your work done properly* |

You can measure your progress about the four quadrants on a monthly basis on a scale of 1 (very good) to 7 (very poor). Always assign 7 points to the area that you are happiest with and other numbers to the remaining quadrants in relation to that one. Afterward, consider whether you want to make any changes to how you are approaching these areas of your life and how you can make those changes. You can also use the spreadsheet you created to manage your worries.

One final point on the topic of stress, even if it may seem trivial: be mindful of your mood, and try to stay upbeat! What you need to do that depends on you. Your mood only partially depends on circumstances. Sometimes simply deciding to be in a good mood can do more than most people realize. Everyone has a load of problems to carry, and it is easier to take it if you commit yourself to a positive outlook.

Do things that excite you as often as possible. Perform activities that contribute to what is most important to you. Is it your family? Then plan an excursion with your family! Is it a sport? Then ask someone to go jogging with you, for example. Consciously take the time to do those things that are close to your heart. Maybe you now object that you do not have time for that and that such self-serving activities would only lead to more stress. Try it out! I bet this qualitatively precious time will not incur losses but help you to mount every day with more tranquility. Plan your activities around what is most important to you in your life. What that means is obviously personal to you! It is your treasure, per se, so you have to dig it out yourself. *Abraham Lincoln* had this to say, to send you on your way: "That some achieve great success is proof to all that others can achieve it as well."

# Summary

Stress can foster lactose intolerance symptoms. Increase your resistance to stress by training to use relaxation techniques, naming fears and worries, developing and noting down solution strategies and adding priorities to them. Make sure you keep your life in the right balance by trading-off between the areas that are important to you. Keep your eye on your goal.

# 2.9   General summary

## 1.  What you are dealing with

If you have a lactose intolerance, lactose in foods can irritate your gut. The symptoms occur because of your body's limited capacity to absorb lactose before it reaches your large intestine, where it causes the discomforts. A lactose intolerance is often chronic but does not cause cancer. In most cases, following a fitting diet reduces the symptoms to an acceptable level.

## 2.  Are you a unique case?

According to the *World Gastroenterology Organisation (WGO)*, up to one billion people have a dietary intolerance or IBS around the globe. In a way, you are lucky, as you can use this book to help you to reduce your symptoms.

## 3.  Good reasons to follow this diet

A lactose intolerance accompanies you for a long time, maybe for the rest of your life. If the diet works, it is far cheaper than medical treatment and sometimes even more efficient. Many medicines also have side effects. If the diet works for you, it will also lead to a general improvement in your wellbeing. You should find that you are ill less often, better able to concentrate, better at fulfilling social obligations, stronger at sports—your new diet can even enhance your love life!

## 4.  Why you want to take the level test

Sensitivities differ in their severity. The fewer dietary restrictions you face, the more you save yourself the effort and can enjoy a more varied selection of food.

## 5.  What you should pay attention to for the diet

Two things: First, adhere to your portion sizes, which you find in the tables in Chapter 3. Thus, only eat as much of lactose containing foods as your enzyme workers can handle. You should keep eating foods containing lactose in tolerable amounts, as cheese contains vital fatty acids. Second, eat in a balanced way see Chapter 2.1.4.

## 6. Dealing with setbacks

You have decided to change your diet and have made the first steps in that direction. Now, you have to stick to it. Moreover, that means to assess properly short-term setbacks. Rebounds are a part of any change process. What is important is that you get back up! The experience of meeting success after facing a blow will strengthen you immensely and ensure that you will be able to get back up even faster next time around. At some point, your experiences and successes will make it a habit for you to persevere and stick to your diet.

It may help you to set a time each Sunday to fill out the symptom test sheet—independent of the other tests. Doing this will remind you of your goal and let you break down the necessary steps toward it on a weekly basis. What is also important is that you become aware of the hurdles you will face. It will be hard to restrict yourself concerning the consumption of some foods that you have come to love. Particularly at the beginning, it will be unnerving to ask for dietary considerations as a dinner guest. Your nutrition plan will be new to others; you may feel criticized for your insistence on maintaining your new eating habits. Explain that you need to do it for the sake of your health. At the same time, express your appreciation for others' support. Moreover, try not giving dietary advice unless someone asks you for it — respecting the eating habits of others. They are more likely to accept yours in turn.

The adversary left for you to face is not standing next to you at the buffet and believes to know better what you can consume. The best captains are always standing ashore. The adversary is in your head and regularly cries "do it as you did it before. Before it was easier!" The influence of our old habits is often greater than we think. After a few days of tenacity, this caller has his big appearance. As soon, as our vigilance is lower he whispers in our ear "This is how you have always done it, and it has always been good, everything else is too exhaustive for you. Simply, show your adversary your weekly symptom test sheet--it works like garlic against vampires. It is the best mean to get rid of old habits, and form new ones! If you always readjust your heading—your diet to your goal, you will come close to it in the end. If you proceed like that, you have a good chance to win against the trigger and old habit imp.

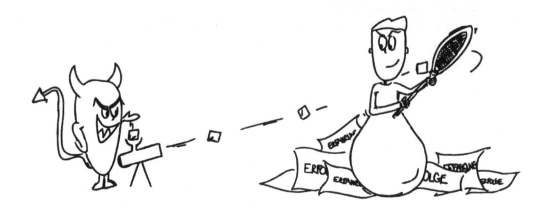

## 7. FAQs

**What do you recommend concerning the diet?** Drink at least 1.5 L of water every day. Eat a variety of foods. Even if you are lactose intolerant, you can try to eat dry cheese (for example) to cover your need for short-chain fatty acids. It is ok to eat foods that contain lactose; they can even be good for you as long as you keep within your restrictions. To do even more for your health, work out regularly.

**What can you do if a drink contains too much of lactose to drink a regular glass full?** By diluting it with water, you can multiply your tolerable portion. Another option is to take the necessary number of lactase enzyme capsules.

**How can you save on cooking time?** Cook larger portion sizes. Usually, it only takes a little longer than preparing small ones, and warming the food up is quick. You can keep rice and potatoes in the fridge for days, for instance. Purchase lockable glass containers to store your food keeping it fresh longer.

**I have acute symptoms, what can I do?** Take a walk and drink up to three liters of drinking water per day.

## 8. The LAXIBA® quickie

Reduce your consumption of milk or use replacement products such as rice milk. Dry cheese like cheddar contains only a little lactose.

Do not start any diet without a proper diagnosis in advance. If you want to do something for your health, in general, stick to the advice see the Chapters starting on pages 39 and 74.

# FEEDBACK

Congratulations, you have mastered the background and strategy chapter. Around the globe, the brand *LAXIBA* represents an improved quality of life in connection with abdominal diseases and stress. Our goal is to offer you scientific solutions that you can implement swiftly to improve your life. To find out about our latest innovations, visit us at *https://laxiba.com* and register for our useletter.

Many improvements make this second edition the gold standard. Each contribution can help to make the book even better in the future. Thus, I am glad to learn about your experiences and your wishes! There are still grey areas, and regularly new foods enter the market that fit our tables well. To deal with the disease, it is important that you adapt your diet to the capacity of your enzyme workers. Therefore, we are interested in any food you are missing.

Would you like to take part in a coaching concerning the implementation of the diet or a workshop on stress management? We will have an offer that suits you. Visit us at *https://laxiba.com*. We look forward to getting to know you. Finally, I wish you prosperity, happiness and an improvement in your quality of life.

Your author,

Jan Stratbucker – *John@Laxiba.com*

# 3

# FOOD TABLES

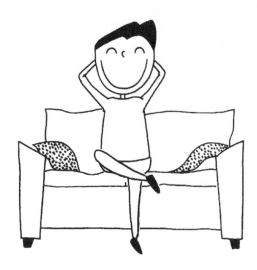

## 3.1   Introduction to the tables

In the following section, you will learn about the tolerable portion sizes for an intolerance towards lactose. The statements all relate to **one meal**, assuming **three meals** per day and that only eat one food containing your trigger. The stated amounts expect you to consume three meals per day, one at roughly 7 am, 1 pm and 7 pm, i.e., each with about **six hours** in between. However, the times are mainly just a reference point just make sure to keep the gaps! If you read the book carefully, you have also learned that eating in between the big meals can have a positive effect on your health. For each food, you can find out how much you can tolerate both in a suitable unit as well as in gram. These statements make cooking as well as eating out easy.

The lists are ordered by category. Milk is listed under beverages-hot beverages, for example. The idea behind this is that you can easily find alternatives, should your tolerated amount be small. At the end of the tables, you also find a food index, though, see page 217, which you can use if you are solely interested in finding out how much of a certain donut you can stomach.

The tables are set up in a manner that is easy to understand. Each page contains about 14 foods. In the tables, you find the category title in the first cell of each table. Below it, you can see the food names and next to them the tolerated amount explained by a proper unit or a smiley. Afterward, you find an explanation as well as the amount in gram. For the first time, you also find the additionally consumable amount per lactase capsule with 12,000 FCC. In the following the symbols and units will be explained further. It is important to us that the data quality is excellent. All figures originate from an analysis conducted by the *University of Minnesota.*

# 3.1.1   Explanation of the symbols

Here you will find an explanation of the symbols. They show you at a glance how many units you can tolerate of the respective food. If you can see a smiley in the list, you will not find an amount. If the smiley looks sad, you should avoid the product if you have a lactose intolerance. If it smiles, you can enjoy it to your heart's content—if there is a big smile, the food is completely free of lactose.

| Symbol | Meaning |
|--------|---------|
| | An average sized potion |
| | Slice(s) |
| | Piece(s) |
| | Hand(s) full |
| | Tablespoon(s) |
| | Bar |
| | Pinch |
| | Cup, 150 ml |
| | Glass, 200 ml |
| | Avoid the consumption. You can tolerate less than ¼ of the lowest amount due to the high lactose load of the food. |
| | Nearly free of lactose. |
| | Free consumption as the food is free of lactose. |

# 3.1.2  Explanation of the statements

| Label | Meaning |
|---|---|
| **Standard amount** | In this column, you find the name of the unit or the meaning of the smiley. Behind it, in brackets, is stated how much gram one unit has followed by the tolerated amount per meal in total. |
| ¼, ½, ¾, 1, 1¼, 1½, 1¾, 2, etc. | The tolerated amount of the respective unit, e.g., "cookie ½ piece" means you tolerate half a cookie of the type per meal, and "soup 1¾ portion" means one and three-fourths of a portion of the soup. |
| Avoid consumption. | Avoid the consumption of the food; it contains much of lactose. |
| Avoid consumption! | Avoid the consumption of the food; it contains very much of lactose. |
| Avoid consumption!! | Avoid the consumption of the food; it contains an extreme load of lactose. |
| **Lactase capsules** | In the last column, you can find the additionally consumable amount per strong, 12,000 FCC, lactase capsule. Important: The additionally consumable amount is independent of your sensitivity level.<br><br>For example, you can find + ¼ for an ice cream. The tolerable amount (stated in the column in front of it) is a ¼ portion, 28g. Now, per lactase capsule you take, you can tolerate ¼ of a portion in addition to the amount your enzyme workers can cover themselves. Doing the math, we get ¼ + ¼, which makes ½ a portion (56g). You can purchase fitting lactase capsules on our homepage, https://laxiba.com. |

# 3.1.3 Your personal sensitivity levels

**Level multiplier and lactose amount per meal by level**

|  | Level | g | Table amount multiplier | Your level |
|---|---|---|---|---|
| Lactose g/meal | 0 | 1.5 | ÷2 | |
| | Standard | 3 | base | |
| | 2 | 6 | ×2 | |
| | 3 | 9 | ×3 | |

**Note:** Please always look at the ingredients as stated on the food packages as well. Especially, if the list does not mention a producer, the composition may vary. In addition, you should consider the weight of one unit in gram. The average portion sizes underlying the statements may be larger or smaller than you expect. For example, 30g of cereals may fill an entire bowl while you can eat 30g of cheesecake in three bites.

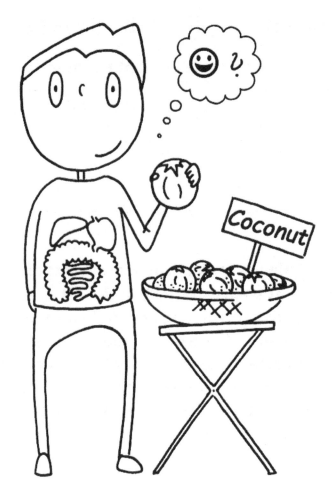

# Check it with the Laxiba App!

1. Get it on the App Store or on Google Play and subscribe

2. Choose "Yes" or your tolerance level for your sensitivities

3. Find the answer with the text or category search option

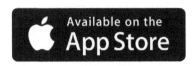
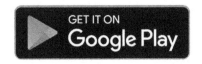

# CATEGORY LIST-INDEX

# 3.2 Athletes

| Athletes | LACTOSE | | Standard amount | |
|---|---|---|---|---|
| Clif Bar®, Chocolate Chip | 9 | | Piece (68g); 612g in total. | +7½ |
| Clif Bar®, Crunchy Peanut Butter | | ☺ | Free of lactose. | |
| Clif Bar®, Oatmeal Raisin Walnut | | ☺ | Free of lactose. | |
| Electrolyte replacement drink | | ☺ | Free of lactose. | |
| Gatorade®, all flavors | 6¼ | | Glass (240g); 1500 mL in total. | +5 |
| Gatorade®, from dry mix, all flavors | | ☺ | Free of lactose. | |
| Glaceau® Vitaminwater 10 | | ☺ | Free of lactose. | |
| Glaceau® Vitaminwater Energy | | ☺ | Free of lactose. | |
| Glaceau® Vitaminwater Essential | | ☺ | Free of lactose. | |
| Glaceau® Vitaminwater Focus | | ☺ | Free of lactose. | |
| Glaceau® Vitaminwater Power-C | | ☺ | Free of lactose. | |
| Glaceau® Vitaminwater Revive | | ☺ | Free of lactose. | |
| High-protein Bar, generic | 39¼ | | Piece (65g); 2551g in total. | +32¾ |
| Power Bar® 20g Protein Plus, Chocolate Crisp | 3 | | Piece (61g); 183g in total. | +2½ |
| Power Bar® 20g Protein Plus, Chocolate Peanut Butter | 3 | | Piece (61g); 183g in total. | +2½ |

| Athletes | LACTOSE | | Standard amount | |
|---|---|---|---|---|
| Power Bar® 30g Protein Plus, Chocolate Brownie | 2 | | Piece (70g); 140g in total. | +1½ |
| Power Bar® Harvest Energy®, Double Chocolate Crisp | 2¾ | | Piece (65g); 179g in total. | +2¼ |
| Power Bar® Performance Energy®, Banana | | | Free of lactose. | |
| Power Bar® Performance Energy®, Chocolate | | | Free of lactose. | |
| Power Bar® Performance Energy®, Cookie Dough | | | Free of lactose. | |
| Power Bar® Performance Energy®, Mixed Berry Blast | | | Free of lactose. | |
| Power Bar® Performance Energy®, Vanilla Crisp | | | Free of lactose. | |
| Powerade®, all flavors | 6¼ | | Glass (240g); 1500 mL in total. | +5 |

# 3.3 Beverages

## 3.3.1 Alcoholic

| Alcoholic | LACTOSE | Standard amount | ⊟ |
|---|---|---|---|
| Ale | ☺ | Free of lactose. | |
| Amaretto | ☺ | Free of lactose. | |
| Apple juice or cider, made from frozen | ☺ | Free of lactose. | |
| Apple juice or cider, unsweetened | ☺ | Free of lactose. | |
| Applejack liquor | ☺ | Free of lactose. | |
| Aquavit | ☺ | Free of lactose. | |
| Beer | ☺ | Free of lactose. | |
| Beer, low alcohol | ☺ | Free of lactose. | |
| Beer, low carb | ☺ | Free of lactose. | |
| Beer, non alcoholic | ☺ | Free of lactose. | |
| Black Russian | ☺ | Free of lactose. | |
| Bloody Mary | ☺ | Free of lactose. | |
| Bourbon | ☺ | Free of lactose. | |
| Brandy | ☺ | Free of lactose. | |

| Alcoholic | LACTOSE | Standard amount | |
|---|---|---|---|
| Burgundy wine, red | 😊 | Free of lactose. | |
| Burgundy wine, white | 😊 | Free of lactose. | |
| Campari® | 😊 | Free of lactose. | |
| Cape Cod | 😊 | Free of lactose. | |
| Champagne punch | 😊 | Free of lactose. | |
| Champagne, white | 😊 | Free of lactose. | |
| Chardonnay | 😊 | Free of lactose. | |
| Club soda | 😊 | Free of lactose. | |
| Cognac | 😊 | Free of lactose. | |
| Cointreau® | 😊 | Free of lactose. | |
| Creme de Cocoa | 😊 | Free of lactose. | |
| Creme de menthe | 😊 | Free of lactose. | |
| Curacao | 😊 | Free of lactose. | |
| Daiquiri | 😊 | Free of lactose. | |
| Eggnog, regular | 🥛 | Glass (240g); Avoid consumption!! | 0.2 |
| Fruit punch, alcoholic | 😊 | Free of lactose. | |

| Alcoholic | LACTOSE | Standard amount | |
|---|---|---|---|
| Gibson | ☺ | Free of lactose. | |
| Gin | ☺ | Free of lactose. | |
| Grand Marnier® | ☺ | Free of lactose. | |
| Grasshopper | 1 🥛 | Glass (240g); 240 mL in total. | +¾ |
| Harvey Wallbanger | ☺ | Free of lactose. | |
| Kamikaze | ☺ | Free of lactose. | |
| Kirsch | ☺ | Free of lactose. | |
| Light beer | ☺ | Free of lactose. | |
| Liqueur, coffee flavored | ☺ | Free of lactose. | |
| Long Island iced tea | ☺ | Free of lactose. | |
| Mai Tai | ☺ | Free of lactose. | |
| Malt liquor | ☺ | Free of lactose. | |
| Manhattan | ☺ | Free of lactose. | |
| Margarita, frozen | ☺ | Free of lactose. | |
| Martini® | ☺ | Free of lactose. | |
| Merlot, red | ☺ | Free of lactose. | |

| Alcoholic | LACTOSE | Standard amount | |
|---|---|---|---|
| Merlot, white | 🙂 | Free of lactose. | |
| Mint Julep | 🙂 | Free of lactose. | |
| Mojito | 🙂 | Free of lactose. | |
| Muscatel | 🙂 | Free of lactose. | |
| Non-alcoholic wine | 🙂 | Free of lactose. | |
| Ouzo | 🙂 | Free of lactose. | |
| Pina colada | 🙂 | Free of lactose. | |
| Port wine | 🙂 | Free of lactose. | |
| Riesling | 🙂 | Free of lactose. | |
| Rob Roy | 🙂 | Free of lactose. | |
| Rompope (eggnog with alcohol) | ¼ | Glass (240g); 60 mL in total. | +¼ |
| Root beer | 🙂 | Free of lactose. | |
| Rose wine, other types | 🙂 | Free of lactose. | |
| Rum | 🙂 | Free of lactose. | |
| Rum and cola | 🙂 | Free of lactose. | |
| Rusty nail | 🙂 | Free of lactose. | |

| Alcoholic | LACTOSE | Standard amount |
|---|---|---|
| Sake | ☺ | Free of lactose. |
| Sambuca | ☺ | Free of lactose. |
| Sangria | ☺ | Free of lactose. |
| Schnapps, all flavors | ☺ | Free of lactose. |
| Scotch and soda | ☺ | Free of lactose. |
| Screwdriver | ☺ | Free of lactose. |
| Seabreeze | ☺ | Free of lactose. |
| Singapore sling | ☺ | Free of lactose. |
| Sloe gin | ☺ | Free of lactose. |
| Sloe gin fizz | ☺ | Free of lactose. |
| Southern Comfort® | ☺ | Free of lactose. |
| Sylvaner | ☺ | Free of lactose. |
| Tequila | ☺ | Free of lactose. |
| Tequila sunrise | ☺ | Free of lactose. |
| Tokaji Wine | ☺ | Free of lactose. |

| Alcoholic | LACTOSE | Standard amount | |
|---|---|---|---|
| Triple Sec | 🙂 | Free of lactose. | |
| Vodka | 🙂 | Free of lactose. | |
| Whiskey | 🙂 | Free of lactose. | |
| Whiskey sour | 🙂 | Free of lactose. | |
| White Russian | 1¼ 🥛 | Glass (240g); 300 mL in total. | +1 |
| Wine spritzer | 🙂 | Free of lactose. | |

## 3.3.2　Hot beverages

| Hot beverages | LACTOSE | Standard amount | |
|---|---|---|---|
| Americano, decaf, without flavored syrup | ☺ | Free of lactose. | |
| Americano, with flavored syrup | ☺ | Free of lactose. | |
| Americano, without flavored syrup | ☺ | Free of lactose. | |
| Brown sugar | ☺ | Free of lactose. | |
| Cafe au lait, without flavored syrup | ½ | Cup (150g); 75 mL in total. | +¼ |
| Cafe latte, with flavored syrup | ½ | Cup (150g); 75 mL in total. | +¼ |
| Cafe latte, without flavored syrup | ½ | Cup (150g); 75 mL in total. | +¼ |
| Camomile tea | ☺ | Free of lactose. | |
| Cappuccino, bottled or canned | ½ | Cup (150g); 75 mL in total. | +½ |
| Cappuccino, decaf, with flavored syrup | ½ | Cup (150g); 75 mL in total. | +¼ |
| Cappuccino, decaf, without flavored syrup | ½ | Cup (150g); 75 mL in total. | +¼ |
| Chai tea | ☺ | Free of lactose. | |
| Chicory coffee | ☺ | Free of lactose. | |
| Coffee substitute, prepared | ☺ | Free of lactose. | |
| Coffee, prepared from flavored mix, sugar free | ☺ | Nearly free of lactose | |

| Hot beverages | LACTOSE | | Standard amount | |
|---|---|---|---|---|
| Dandelion tea | | 😊 | Free of lactose. | |
| Demitasse | | 😊 | Free of lactose. | |
| Dove® Promises, Milk Chocolate | ¼ | ☕ | Cup (150g); 38 mL in total. | 0.22 |
| Earl Grey, strong | | 😊 | Free of lactose. | |
| Espresso, without flavored syrup | | 😊 | Free of lactose. | |
| Evaporated milk, diluted, skim (fat free) | ¼ | ☕ | Cup (150g); 38 mL in total. | +¼ |
| Fennel tea | | 😊 | Free of lactose. | |
| Frappuccino® | ½ | ☕ | Cup (150g); 75 mL in total. | +½ |
| Frappuccino®, bottled or canned | ½ | ☕ | Cup (150g); 75 mL in total. | +½ |
| Frappuccino®, bottled or canned, light | ½ | ☕ | Cup (150g); 75 mL in total. | +½ |
| Green tea, strong | | 😊 | Free of lactose. | |
| Herbal tea | | 😊 | Free of lactose. | |
| Hershey's® Bliss Hot Drink White Chocolate, prepared | ¼ | ☕ | Cup (150g); 38 mL in total. | +¼ |
| Hot chocolate, homemade | ¼ | ☕ | Cup (150g); 38 mL in total. | +¼ |
| Instant coffee mix, unprepared | | 😊 | Free of lactose. | |
| Irish coffee with alcohol and whipped cream | 3¾ | ☕ | Cup (150g); 563 mL in total. | +3 |

| Hot beverages | LACTOSE | | Standard amount | |
|---|---|---|---|---|
| Jasmine tea | | ☺ | Free of lactose. | |
| Light cream | 5¼ | | Portion (15g); 79g in total. | +4½ |
| Milk, lactose reduced Lactaid®, skim (fat free) | | ☺ | Free of lactose. | |
| Milk, lactose reduced Lactaid®, whole | | ☺ | Free of lactose. | |
| Milk, unprepared dry powder, nonfat, instant | ¼ | | Portion (22.64g); 6g in total. | 0.22 |
| Mocha, without flavored syrup | ½ | | Cup (150g); 75 mL in total. | +¼ |
| Nestle® Hot Cocoa Dark Chocolate, prepared | ¼ | | Cup (150g); 38 mL in total. | +¼ |
| Nestle® Hot Cocoa Rich Milk Chocolate, prepared | ¼ | | Cup (150g); 38 mL in total. | +¼ |
| Oolong tea | | ☺ | Free of lactose. | |
| Soy milk, chocolate, sweetened with sugar, not fortified | | ☺ | Free of lactose. | |
| Splenda® | | ☺ | Free of lactose. | |
| Starbucks® Hot Cocoa Double Chocolate, prepared | ¼ | | Cup (150g); 38 mL in total. | +¼ |
| Starbucks® Hot Cocoa Salted Caramel, prepared | ¼ | | Cup (150g); 38 mL in total. | +¼ |
| Sugar, white granulated | | ☺ | Free of lactose. | |
| Sweetened condensed milk | ½ | | Portion (38g); 19g in total. | +½ |
| Sweetened condensed milk, reduced fat | ½ | | Portion (39g); 20g in total. | +½ |

| Hot beverages | LACTOSE | | Standard amount | |
|---|---|---|---|---|
| Swiss Miss® Hot Cocoa Sensible Sweets Diet, sugar free, prepared | ¼ | | Cup (150g); 38 mL in total. | +¼ |
| Whipped cream, aerosol | | | Nearly free of lactose | |
| Whipped cream, aerosol, fat free | 18¾ | | Portion (5g); 94g in total. | +15¾ |
| White tea | | | Free of lactose. | |
| Zsweet® | | | Free of lactose. | |

# 3.3.3   Juices

| Juices | LACTOSE | Standard amount | |
|---|---|---|---|
| Apple banana strawberry juice | 😊 | Free of lactose. | |
| Apple grape juice | 😊 | Free of lactose. | |
| Apricot nectar | 😊 | Free of lactose. | |
| Arby's® orange juice | 😊 | Free of lactose. | |
| Black cherry juice | 😊 | Free of lactose. | |
| Black currant juice | 😊 | Free of lactose. | |
| Blackberry juice | 😊 | Free of lactose. | |
| Capri Sun®, all flavors | 😊 | Free of lactose. | |
| Carrot juice | 😊 | Free of lactose. | |
| Cranberry juice cocktail, with apple juice | 😊 | Free of lactose. | |
| Cranberry juice cocktail, with blueberry juice | 😊 | Free of lactose. | |
| Fruit drink or punch, ready to drink | 😊 | Free of lactose. | |
| Grapefruit juice, unsweetened, white | 😊 | Free of lactose. | |
| Kern's® Mango-Orange Nectar | 😊 | Free of lactose. | |
| Kern's® Strawberry Nectar | 😊 | Free of lactose. | |

| Juices | LACTOSE | Standard amount | |
|---|---|---|---|
| Lemon juice, fresh | ☺ | Free of lactose. | |
| Libby's® Apricot Nectar | ☺ | Free of lactose. | |
| Libby's® Banana Nectar | ☺ | Free of lactose. | |
| Libby's® Juicy Juice®, Apple Grape | ☺ | Free of lactose. | |
| Libby's® Juicy Juice®, Grape | ☺ | Free of lactose. | |
| Libby's® Pear Nectar | ☺ | Free of lactose. | |
| Lime juice, fresh | ☺ | Free of lactose. | |
| Mango nectar | ☺ | Free of lactose. | |
| Northland® Cranberry Juice, all flavors | ☺ | Free of lactose. | |
| Orange kiwi passion juice | ☺ | Free of lactose. | |
| Passion fruit juice | ☺ | Free of lactose. | |
| Peach juice | ☺ | Free of lactose. | |
| Pear juice | ☺ | Free of lactose. | |
| Pineapple juice | ☺ | Free of lactose. | |
| Pineapple orange drink | ☺ | Free of lactose. | |
| Pomegranate juice | ☺ | Free of lactose. | |

| Juices | LACTOSE | Standard amount | |
|---|---|---|---|
| Raspberry juice | ☺ | Free of lactose. | |
| Tomato juice | ☺ | Free of lactose. | |
| V-8® 100% A-C-E Vitamin Rich Vegetable Juice | ☺ | Free of lactose. | |
| Veryfine Cranberry Raspberry | ☺ | Free of lactose. | |

# 3.3.4 Other beverages

| Other beverages | LACTOSE | Standard amount | |
|---|---|---|---|
| 7 UP® | 🙂 | Free of lactose. | |
| Canfield's® Root Beer | 🙂 | Free of lactose. | |
| Canfield's® Root Beer, diet | 🙂 | Free of lactose. | |
| Cherry Coke® | 🙂 | Free of lactose. | |
| Coke Zero® | 🙂 | Free of lactose. | |
| Coke® | 🙂 | Free of lactose. | |
| Coke® with Lime | 🙂 | Free of lactose. | |
| Diet 7 UP® | 🙂 | Free of lactose. | |
| Diet Coke® | 🙂 | Free of lactose. | |
| Diet Dr. Pepper® | 🙂 | Free of lactose. | |
| Diet Pepsi®, fountain | 🙂 | Free of lactose. | |
| Fanta Zero®, fruit flavors | 🙂 | Free of lactose. | |
| Fanta® Red | 🙂 | Free of lactose. | |
| Fanta®, fruit flavors | 🙂 | Free of lactose. | |
| Ginger ale | 🙂 | Free of lactose. | |

| Other beverages | LACTOSE | Standard amount |
|---|---|---|
| Lipton® Iced Tea Mix, sweetened with sugar, prepared | 🙂 | Free of lactose. |
| Lipton® Instant 100% Tea, unsweetened, prepared | 🙂 | Free of lactose. |
| Mineral Water | 🙂 | Free of lactose. |
| Monster® Energy® | 🙂 | Free of lactose. |
| Monster® Khaos | 🙂 | Free of lactose. |
| Mountain Dew® | 🙂 | Free of lactose. |
| Mountain Dew® Code Red | 🙂 | Free of lactose. |
| Nestea® 100% Tea, unsweetened, dry | 🙂 | Free of lactose. |
| Nestea® Iced Tea, Sugar Free, dry | 🙂 | Free of lactose. |
| Nestea® Iced Tea, Sugar Free, prepared | 🙂 | Free of lactose. |
| Nestea® Iced Tea, sweetened with sugar, dry | 🙂 | Free of lactose. |
| No Fear® | 🙂 | Free of lactose. |
| No Fear® Sugar Free | 🙂 | Free of lactose. |
| Pepsi® | 🙂 | Free of lactose. |
| Pepsi® Max | 🙂 | Free of lactose. |
| Pepsi® Twist | 🙂 | Free of lactose. |

| Other beverages | LACTOSE | Standard amount |
|---|---|---|
| Red Bull® Energy Drink | ☺ | Free of lactose. |
| Red Bull® Energy Drink Sugar Free | ☺ | Free of lactose. |
| Rockstar Original® | ☺ | Free of lactose. |
| Rockstar Original® Sugar Free | ☺ | Free of lactose. |
| Schweppes® Bitter Lemon | ☺ | Free of lactose. |
| Spearmint tea | ☺ | Free of lactose. |
| Sprite® | ☺ | Free of lactose. |
| Sprite® Zero | ☺ | Free of lactose. |
| Tap water | ☺ | Free of lactose. |
| Tonic water | ☺ | Free of lactose. |
| Tonic water, diet | ☺ | Free of lactose. |
| Vanilla Coke® | ☺ | Free of lactose. |
| Yerba® Mate tea | ☺ | Free of lactose. |

# 3.4  Cold dishes

## 3.4.1  Bread

| Bread | LACTOSE | Standard amount | |
|---|---|---|---|
| Baguette | 🙂 | Free of lactose. | |
| Cracked wheat bread, with raisins | 🙂 | Free of lactose. | |
| English muffin bread | 🙂 | Free of lactose. | |
| Focaccia bread | 🙂 | Free of lactose. | |
| French or Vienna roll | 🙂 | Free of lactose. | |
| GG® Scandinavian Bran Crispbread (Health Valley®) | 🙂 | Free of lactose. | |
| Gluten free bread | 🙂 | Free of lactose. | |
| Newman's Own® Organic Pretzels, Spelt | 🙂 | Free of lactose. | |
| Potato bread | 6¼ | Slice (34g); 213g in total. | +5¼ |
| Pumpernickel roll | 🙂 | Free of lactose. | |
| Rice bread | 🙂 | Free of lactose. | |
| Rye bread | 🙂 | Free of lactose. | |
| Rye roll | 🙂 | Free of lactose. | |
| Sourdough bread | 🙂 | Free of lactose. | |

| Bread | LACTOSE | Standard amount | |
|---|---|---|---|
| Soy bread | 3½ | Slice (42g); 147g in total. | +3 |
| Toast, cinnamon and sugar, whole wheat bread | 49½ | Slice (42g); 2079g in total. | +41¼ |
| Toast, wheat bread, with butter | 62½ | Slice (42g); 2625g in total. | +52 |
| Triticale bread | | Free of lactose. | |
| White bread, store bought | | Nearly free of lactose | |
| White whole grain wheat bread | | Free of lactose. | |
| Whole wheat bread, store bought | | Free of lactose. | |

# 3.4.2 Cereals

| Cereals | LACTOSE | Standard amount | |
|---|---|---|---|
| All-Bran® Original (Kellogg's®) | 😊 | Free of lactose. | |
| Amaranth Flakes (Arrowhead Mills) | 😊 | Free of lactose. | |
| Cascadian Farm® Organic Gran. Bar, Dark Chocolate Cranberry | 10 🍰 | Piece (35g); 350g in total. | +8¼ |
| Cheerios® Snack Mix, all flavors | 😊 | Free of lactose. | |
| Chocolate Chex® (General Mills®) | 😊 | Free of lactose. | |
| Cinnamon toast crunch® (General Mills®) | 😊 | Free of lactose. | |
| Cinnamon Toasters® (Malt-O-Meal®) | 😊 | Free of lactose. | |
| Cocoa Krispies® (Kellogg's®) | 😊 | Free of lactose. | |
| Cocoa Puffs® (General Mills®) | 😊 | Free of lactose. | |
| Corn Chex® (General Mills®) | 😊 | Free of lactose. | |
| Corn Flakes (Kellogg's®) | 😊 | Free of lactose. | |
| Crunchy Nut Roasted Nut & Honey (Kellogg's®) | 🙂 | Nearly free of lactose | |
| Essentials Oat Bran cereal (Quaker®) | 😊 | Free of lactose. | |
| Evaporated milk, diluted, skim (fat free) | 🥛 | Glass (240g); Avoid consumption!! | 0.19 |
| Familia Swiss Muesli®, Original Recipe | 😊 | Free of lactose. | |

| Cereals | LACTOSE | Standard amount | ⊕ |
|---|---|---|---|
| Fiber One Original® (General Mills®) | 😊 | Free of lactose. | |
| Fiber One® Nutty Clusters & Almonds (General Mills®) | 😊 | Free of lactose. | |
| Froot Loops® (Kellogg's®) | 😊 | Free of lactose. | |
| Frosted Flakes® (Kellogg's®) | 😊 | Free of lactose. | |
| Frosted Flakes® Reduced Sugar (Kellogg's®) | 😊 | Free of lactose. | |
| Frosted Mini-Wheats Big Bite® (Kellogg's®) | 😊 | Free of lactose. | |
| GoLEAN® Crisp! Cereal, Cinnamon Crumble (Kashi®) | 😊 | Free of lactose. | |
| GoLEAN® Crunch! Cereal, Honey Almond Flax (Kashi®) | 😊 | Free of lactose. | |
| Health Valley® Multigrain Chewy Granola Bar, Chocolate Chip | 12 🍰 | Piece (29g); 348g in total. | +10 |
| Honey | 🙂 | Nearly free of lactose | |
| Honey Nut Chex® (General Mills®) | 🙂 | Free of lactose. | |
| Honey Smacks® (Kellogg's®) | 🙂 | Free of lactose. | |
| Kashi® Chewy Granola Bar, Cherry Dark Chocolate | 10 🍰 | Piece (35g); 350g in total. | +8¼ |
| Maple syrup, pure | 🙂 | Free of lactose. | |
| Milk, lactose reduced Lactaid®, skim (fat free) fortified with calcium or not | 🙂 | Free of lactose. | |

| Cereals | LACTOSE | Standard amount | |
|---|---|---|---|
| Mueslix® (Kellogg's®) | ☺ | Free of lactose. | |
| Rice Krispies® (Kellogg's®) | ☺ | Free of lactose. | |
| Sorghum | ☺ | Free of lactose. | |
| Special K® Blueberry cereal (Kellogg's®) | ☺ | Free of lactose. | |
| Special K® Cinnamon Pecan cereal (Kellogg's®) | ☺ | Free of lactose. | |
| Special K® Original cereal (Kellogg's®) | 13 | Portion (30g); 390g in total. | +10¾ |
| Special K® Red Berries cereal (Kellogg's®) | ☺ | Free of lactose. | |
| Sprinkles Cookie Crisp® (General Mills®) | ☺ | Free of lactose. | |
| Sunbelt Bakery® Chewy Granola Bar, Banana Harvest | 14 | Piece (25g); 350g in total. | +11¾ |
| Sunbelt Bakery® Chewy Granola Bar, Blueberry Harvest | 14 | Piece (25g); 350g in total. | +11¾ |
| Sunbelt Bakery® Chewy Granola Bar, Golden Almond | 4 | Piece (28g); 112g in total. | +3¼ |
| Sunbelt Bakery® Chewy Granola Bar, Low Fat Oatmeal Raisin | 11¾ | Piece (30g); 353g in total. | +9¾ |
| Sunbelt Bakery® Chewy Granola Bar, Oats & Honey | 13 | Piece (27g); 351g in total. | +10¾ |
| Sunbelt Bakery® Fudge Dipped Chewy Granola Bar, Coconut | 12 | Piece (29g); 348g in total. | +10 |
| Weetabix® Organic Crispy Flakes&Fiber Barbara's Bakery® | ☺ | Free of lactose. | |
| Wheaties® (General Mills®) | ☺ | Free of lactose. | |

## 3.4.3 Cold cut

| Cold cut | LACTOSE | | Standard amount | |
|---|---|---|---|---|
| Almond butter, salted | | 😊 | Free of lactose. | |
| Almond butter, unsalted | | 😊 | Free of lactose. | |
| Alpine Lace 25% Reduced Fat, Mozzarella | 37¼ | 🍲 | Portion (30g); 1118g in total. | +31 |
| American cheese, processed | 4½ | 🍲 | Portion (30g); 135g in total. | +3¾ |
| Blue cheese | 20 | 🍲 | Portion (30g); 600g in total. | +16½ |
| Bologna, beef ring | | 😊 | Free of lactose. | |
| Bologna, combination of meats, light (reduced fat) | | 😊 | Free of lactose. | |
| Brie cheese | 22 | 🍲 | Portion (30g); 660g in total. | +18½ |
| Butter, light, salted | | 🙂 | Nearly free of lactose | |
| Butter, unsalted | | 🙂 | Nearly free of lactose | |
| Camembert cheese | 21½ | 🍲 | Portion (30g); 645g in total. | +18 |
| Cheddar cheese, natural | 43¼ | 🍲 | Portion (30g); 1298g in total. | +36 |
| Cheese sauce, store bought | ¼ | 🍲 | Portion (66g); 17g in total. | +¼ |
| Colby Jack cheese | 27¼ | 🍲 | Portion (30g); 818g in total. | +22¾ |
| Cottage cheese, 1% fat, lactose reduced | 3¼ | 🍲 | Portion (110g); 358g in total. | +2¾ |

| Cold cut | LACTOSE | | Standard amount | |
|---|---|---|---|---|
| Cottage cheese, uncreamed dry curd | 3½ | | Portion (55g); 193g in total. | +2¾ |
| Cream cheese spread | 2¾ | | Portion (30g); 83g in total. | +2¼ |
| Cream cheese, whipped, flavored | 2½ | | Portion (30g); 75g in total. | +2 |
| Cream cheese, whipped, plain | 3 | | Portion (30g); 90g in total. | +2½ |
| Edam cheese | 6¾ | | Portion (30g); 203g in total. | +5¾ |
| Fleischmann's® Move Over Butter Margarine, tub, whipped | 21¾ | | Portion (9g); 196g in total. | +18 |
| Goat cheese, hard | 4½ | | Portion (30g); 135g in total. | +3¾ |
| Gorgonzola cheese | 20 | | Portion (30g); 600g in total. | +16½ |
| Gouda cheese | 4½ | | Portion (30g); 135g in total. | +3¾ |
| Honey | | | Nearly free of lactose | |
| Hot dog, combination of meats, plain | | | Free of lactose. | |
| Jam or preserves | | | Free of lactose. | |
| Jam or preserves, reduced sugar | | | Free of lactose. | |
| Jam or preserves, sugar free with aspartame | | | Free of lactose. | |
| Jam or preserves, sugar free with saccharin | | | Free of lactose. | |
| Jam or preserves, sugar free with sucralose | | | Free of lactose. | |

| Cold cut | LACTOSE | Standard amount | 🙂 |
|---|---|---|---|
| Jam or preserves, without sugar or artificial sweetener | | Free of lactose. | |
| Kraft® Cheese Spread, Roka Blue | 1¾ | Portion (30g); 53g in total. | +1¼ |
| Limburger cheese | 20¼ | Portion (30g); 608g in total. | +17 |
| Maple syrup, pure | | Free of lactose. | |
| Margarine, diet, fat free | 15½ | Portion (14g); 217g in total. | +13 |
| Margarine, tub, salted, sunflower oil | 30 | Portion (14.19g); 426g in total. | +25 |
| Marmalade, sugar free with aspartame | | Free of lactose. | |
| Marmalade, sugar free with saccharin | | Free of lactose. | |
| Marmalade, sugar free with sucralose | | Free of lactose. | |
| Mascarpone | 2½ | Portion (30g); 75g in total. | +2 |
| Mortadella | | Free of lactose. | |
| Muenster cheese, natural | 8¾ | Portion (30g); 263g in total. | +7¼ |
| Nutella® (filbert spread) | 32¼ | Portion (37g); 1193g in total. | +27 |
| Roquefort cheese | 5 | Portion (30g); 150g in total. | +4 |
| Smart Balance® Light with Flax Oil Margarine, tub | 32¼ | Portion (14g); 452g in total. | +27 |
| Smart Balance® Margarine | 31 | Portion (14g); 434g in total. | +25¾ |

| Cold cut | LACTOSE | | Standard amount | |
|---|---|---|---|---|
| Soy Kaas Fat Free, all flavors | 9 | | Portion (30g); 270g in total. | +7½ |
| Swiss cheese, natural | | ☺ | Nearly free of lactose | |
| Swiss cheese, natural, low sodium | | ☺ | Nearly free of lactose | |
| Tilsit cheese | 5¼ | | Portion (30g); 158g in total. | +4¼ |

## 3.4.4 Dairy products

| Dairy products | LACTOSE | | Standard amount | |
|---|---|---|---|---|
| Almond milk, vanilla or other flavors, unsweetened | | 😊 | Free of lactose. | |
| Breyers® Light! Boosts Immunity Yogurt, all flavors | ½ | 🍰 | Piece (115g); 58g in total. | +¼ |
| Breyers® No Sugar Added Ice Cream, Vanilla | 3¼ | 🥄 | Tbsp. (15g); 49g in total. | +2½ |
| Breyers® YoCrunch Light Nonfat Yogurt, with granola | ¼ | 🍰 | Piece (250g); 63g in total. | 0.24 |
| Cabot® Non Fat Yogurt, plain | ¼ | 🍰 | Piece (150g); 38g in total. | 0.22 |
| Cabot® Non Fat Yogurt, vanilla | ¼ | 🍰 | Piece (150g); 38g in total. | +¼ |
| Chobani® Nonfat Greek Yogurt, Black Cherry | 5¼ | 🥄 | Tbsp. (15g); 79g in total. | +4½ |
| Chobani® Nonfat Greek Yogurt, Lemon | ½ | 🍰 | Piece (150g); 75g in total. | +¼ |
| Chobani® Nonfat Greek Yogurt, Peach | ¼ | 🍰 | Piece (250g); 63g in total. | +¼ |
| Chobani® Nonfat Greek Yogurt, Raspberry | ¼ | 🍰 | Piece (250g); 63g in total. | +¼ |
| Chobani® Nonfat Greek Yogurt, Strawberry | ¼ | 🍰 | Piece (250g); 63g in total. | +¼ |
| Chocolate pudding, store bought | ¾ | 🍰 | Piece (200g); 150g in total. | +½ |
| Chocolate pudding, store bought, sugar free | 89¼ | 🥄 | Tbsp. (15g); 1339g in total. | +74¼ |
| Cottage cheese, uncreamed dry curd | 3½ | 🥣 | Portion (55g); 193g in total. | +2¾ |

| Dairy products | LACTOSE | | Standard amount | |
|---|---|---|---|---|
| Dannon® Activia® Light Yogurt, vanilla | ¼ | | Piece (115g); 29g in total. | +¼ |
| Dannon® Activia® Yogurt, plain | ½ | | Piece (115g); 58g in total. | +¼ |
| Dannon® Greek Yogurt, Honey | ½ | | Piece (150g); 75g in total. | +¼ |
| Dannon® Greek Yogurt, Plain | ½ | | Piece (150g); 75g in total. | +¼ |
| Dannon® la Crème Yogurt, fruit flavors | ¼ | | Piece (115g); 29g in total. | +¼ |
| Evaporated milk, diluted, 2% fat (reduced fat) | | | Glass (240g); Avoid consumption!! | 0.19 |
| Evaporated milk, diluted, skim (fat free) | | | Glass (240g); Avoid consumption!! | 0.19 |
| Evaporated milk, diluted, whole | | | Glass (240g); Avoid consumption!! | 0.2 |
| Feta cheese | 2¼ | | Portion (30g); 68g in total. | +2 |
| Feta cheese, fat free | ¾ | | Portion (30g); 23g in total. | +¾ |
| Fondue sauce | | | Nearly free of lactose | |
| GO Veggie!™ Rice Slices, all flavors | 12 | | Portion (30g); 360g in total. | +10 |
| Greek yogurt, plain, nonfat, | ¼ | | Piece (250g); 63g in total. | +¼ |
| Half and half | 2¼ | | Portion (30g); 68g in total. | +1¾ |
| Kefir | ¼ | | Portion (220g); 55g in total. | +¼ |
| Laughing Cow® Mini Babybel®, Cheddar | | | Nearly free of lactose | |

| Dairy products | LACTOSE | | Standard amount | 🌡 |
|---|---|---|---|---|
| Laughing Cow® Mini Babybel®, Original | 12¾ | | Piece (21g); 268g in total. | +10½ |
| Licuado, mango | ¼ | | Glass (240g); 60 mL in total. | +¼ |
| Light cream | 5¼ | | Portion (15g); 79g in total. | +4½ |
| Milk, lactose reduced Lactaid®, skim (fat free) | | ☺ | Free of lactose. | |
| Milk, lactose reduced Lactaid®, whole | | ☺ | Free of lactose. | |
| Milk, lactose reduced, skim (fat free), with calcium Lactaid® | | ☺ | Free of lactose. | |
| Mozzarella cheese, fat free | 2¾ | | Portion (30g); 83g in total. | +2¼ |
| Mozzarella cheese, whole milk | 2¾ | | Portion (30g); 83g in total. | +2¼ |
| Oat milk | | ☺ | Free of lactose. | |
| Parmesan cheese, dry (grated) | | ☺ | Nearly free of lactose | |
| Parmesan cheese, dry (grated), nonfat | | ☺ | Nearly free of lactose | +75¾ |
| Pudding mix, other flavors, cooked type | | ☺ | Free of lactose. | |
| Rice milk, plain or original, unsweetened, enriched, ready | | ☺ | Free of lactose. | |
| Rice pudding (arroz con leche), coconut, raisins | ½ | | Piece (200g); 100g in total. | +¼ |
| Rice pudding (arroz con leche), plain | ½ | | Piece (200g); 100g in total. | +¼ |
| Rice pudding (arroz con leche), raisins | ½ | | Piece (200g); 100g in total. | +¼ |

| Dairy products | LACTOSE | | Standard amount | |
|---|---|---|---|---|
| Ricotta cheese, part skim milk | 17½ | | Portion (55g); 963g in total. | +14½ |
| Slim-Fast® Easy to Digest, Vanilla, ready-to-drink can | 2 | | Glass (240g); 480 mL in total. | +1¾ |
| Sour cream | 3¼ | | Portion (30g); 98g in total. | +2¾ |
| Soy milk, plain or original, with artificial sweetener, ready | | | Free of lactose. | |
| Soy milk, vanilla or other flavors, sugar, fat free, ready | | | Free of lactose. | |
| Stonyfield® Oikos Greek Yogurt, Blueberry | ¼ | | Piece (250g); 63g in total. | +¼ |
| Stonyfield® Oikos Greek Yogurt, Caramel | ½ | | Piece (100g); 50g in total. | +½ |
| Stonyfield® Oikos Greek Yogurt, Chocolate | ½ | | Piece (150g); 75g in total. | +¼ |
| Stonyfield® Oikos Greek Yogurt, Strawberry | ¼ | | Piece (250g); 63g in total. | +¼ |
| Strawberry milk, plain, prepared | ¼ | | Glass (240g); 60 mL in total. | 0.22 |
| Sweetened condensed milk | ½ | | Portion (38g); 19g in total. | +½ |
| Sweetened condensed milk, reduced fat | ½ | | Portion (39g); 20g in total. | +½ |
| Tofu, raw (not silken), cooked, low fat | | | Free of lactose. | |
| Whipped cream, aerosol | | | Nearly free of lactose | |
| Whipped cream, aerosol, chocolate | 9¾ | | Portion (5g); 49g in total. | +8 |
| Whipped cream, aerosol, fat free | 18¾ | | Portion (5g); 94g in total. | +15¾ |

| Dairy products | LACTOSE | | Standard amount | |
|---|---|---|---|---|
| Yogurt, chocolate or coffee flavors, nonfat, with aspartame | 4 | | Tbsp. (15g); 60g in total. | +3¼ |
| Yogurt, chocolate or coffee flavors, whole milk, sucralose | ¼ | | Piece (250g); 63g in total. | +¼ |
| Yogurt, fruited, whole milk | 2¾ | | Tbsp. (15g); 41g in total. | +2¼ |

## 3.4.5 Nuts and snacks

| Nuts and snacks | LACTOSE | Standard amount |
|---|---|---|
| Almonds, raw | ☺ | Free of lactose. |
| Baby food, zwieback | ☺ | Free of lactose. |
| Brazil nuts, unsalted | ☺ | Free of lactose. |
| Caramel or sugar coated popcorn, store bought | ☺ | Nearly free of lactose |
| Cashews, raw | ☺ | Free of lactose. |
| Cheese cracker | ☺ | Free of lactose. |
| Chestnuts, roasted | ☺ | Free of lactose. |
| Chia seeds | ☺ | Free of lactose. |
| Coconut cream (liquid from grated meat) | ☺ | Free of lactose. |
| Coconut milk, fresh (liquid from grated meat, water added) | ☺ | Free of lactose. |
| Coconut, dried, shredded or flaked, unsweetened | ☺ | Free of lactose. |
| Coconut, fresh | ☺ | Free of lactose. |
| Doritos® Tortilla Chips, Nacho Cheese | ☺ | Nearly free of lactose |
| Filberts, raw | ☺ | Free of lactose. |
| Flax seeds, not fortified | ☺ | Free of lactose. |

| Nuts and snacks | LACTOSE | Standard amount | |
|---|---|---|---|
| Ginko nuts, dried | 😊 | Free of lactose. | |
| Hickorynuts | 😊 | Free of lactose. | |
| Lay's® Potato Chips, Classic | 😊 | Free of lactose. | |
| Lay's® Potato Chips, Salt & Vinegar | 😊 | Free of lactose. | |
| Lay's® Potato Chips, Sour Cream & Onion | 😊 | Free of lactose. | |
| Lay's® Stax Potato Crisps, Cheddar | 😊 | Free of lactose. | |
| Lay's® Stax Potato Crisps, Hot 'n Spicy Barbecue | 😊 | Free of lactose. | |
| Macadamia nuts, raw | 😊 | Free of lactose. | |
| Melba Toast®, Classic (Old London®) | 😊 | Free of lactose. | |
| Old Dutch® Crunch Curls | 4 | Hand (21g); 84g in total. | +3¼ |
| Peanut butter, unsalted | 😊 | Free of lactose. | |
| Peanuts, dry roasted, salted | 😊 | Free of lactose. | |
| Pine nuts, pignolias | 😊 | Free of lactose. | |
| Pistachio nuts, raw | 😊 | Free of lactose. | |
| Poore Brothers® Potato Chips, Salt & Cracked Pepper | 😊 | Free of lactose. | |
| Potato chips, salted | 😊 | Free of lactose. | |

| Nuts and snacks | LACTOSE | Standard amount | |
|---|---|---|---|
| Potato sticks | 😊 | Free of lactose. | |
| Pretzels, hard, unsalted, sticks | 😊 | Free of lactose. | |
| Pringles® Light Fat Free Potato Crisps, Barbecue | 😊 | Free of lactose. | |
| Pringles® Potato Crisps, Loaded Baked Potato | 😊 | Free of lactose. | |
| Pringles® Potato Crisps, Original | 😊 | Free of lactose. | |
| Pringles® Potato Crisps, Salt & Vinegar | 😊 | Free of lactose. | |
| Pumpkin or squash seeds, shelled, unsalted | 😊 | Free of lactose. | |
| Rice cake | 😊 | Free of lactose. | |
| Ritz Cracker (Nabisco®) | 😊 | Free of lactose. | |
| Sesame sticks | 😊 | Free of lactose. | |
| Soy chips | 5¼ | Hand (21g); 110g in total. | +4¼ |
| Sunflower seeds, raw | 😊 | Free of lactose. | |
| Taco John's® nachos | 28 | Hand (21g); 588g in total. | +23¼ |
| Tortilla, white, store bought, fried | 😊 | Free of lactose. | |
| Walnuts | 😊 | Free of lactose. | |
| Wise Onion Flavored Rings | 😊 | Free of lactose. | |

# 3.4.6   Sweet pastries

| Sweet pastries | LACTOSE | | Standard amount | |
|---|---|---|---|---|
| Almond cookies | | ☺ | Nearly free of lactose | |
| Apple cake, glazed | | ☺ | Free of lactose. | |
| Apple strudel | | ☺ | Nearly free of lactose | |
| Archway® Ginger Snaps | | ☺ | Free of lactose. | |
| Archway® Oatmeal Raisin Cookies | 23¾ | 🍰 | Piece (26g); 618g in total. | +19¾ |
| Archway® Peanut Butter Cookies | 23¾ | 🍰 | Piece (34g); 808g in total. | +19¾ |
| Biscotti, chocolate, nuts | | ☺ | Nearly free of lactose | |
| Brownie, chocolate, fat free | 3 | 🍰 | Piece (44g); 132g in total. | +2½ |
| Butter cracker | | ☺ | Free of lactose. | |
| Carrot cake, glazed, homemade | | ☺ | Free of lactose. | |
| Cheesecake, plain or flavored, graham cracker crust, homemade | ½ | 🍰 | Piece (220g); 110g in total. | +½ |
| Cherry pie, bottom crust only | | ☺ | Free of lactose. | |
| Chips Ahoy!® Chewy Gooey Caramel Cookies (Nabisco®) | 12¼ | 🍰 | Piece (15.5g); 190g in total. | +10¼ |
| Chocolate cake, glazed, store bought | | ☺ | Free of lactose. | |

| Sweet pastries | LACTOSE | Standard amount | |
|---|---|---|---|
| Chocolate chip cookies, store bought | ☺ | Free of lactose. | |
| Chocolate cookies, iced, store bought | ☺ | Free of lactose. | |
| Chocolate sandwich cookies, double filling | ☺ | Free of lactose. | |
| Chocolate sandwich cookies, sugar free | ☺ | Nearly free of lactose | |
| Cinnamon crispas (fried flour tortilla, cinnamon, sugar) | ☺ | Free of lactose. | |
| Crepe, plain | 1¼ | Piece (55g); 69g in total. | +1 |
| Croissant, chocolate | 3½ | Piece (69g); 242g in total. | +3 |
| Croissant, fruit | 3½ | Piece (74g); 259g in total. | +3 |
| Danish pastry, frosted or glazed, with cheese filling | 3 | Piece (125g); 375g in total. | +2½ |
| Dare Breaktime Ginger Cookies | ☺ | Free of lactose. | |
| Dare® Lemon Crème Cookies | 32½ | Piece (19.5g); 634g in total. | +27 |
| Doughnut, raised, glazed, coconut topping | 4¾ | Piece (79g); 375g in total. | +4 |
| Doughnut, raised, glazed, plain | 4¾ | Piece (77g); 366g in total. | +4 |
| Doughnut, raised, sugared | 4¾ | Piece (72.5g); 344g in total. | +4 |
| EGG® bread roll | 5¼ | Piece (35g); 184g in total. | +4¼ |
| Elephant ear (crispy) | 4¼ | Piece (59g); 251g in total. | +3½ |

| Sweet pastries | LACTOSE | | Standard amount | ⊖ |
|---|---|---|---|---|
| English muffin, whole wheat, with raisins | 1¼ | | Piece (66g); 83g in total. | +1 |
| French toast, homemade, French bread | 1¼ | | Piece (131g); 164g in total. | +1 |
| Frozen custard, chocolate or coffee flavors | ½ | | Portion (87.5g); 44g in total. | +¼ |
| German chocolate cake, glazed, homemade | | | Free of lactose. | |
| Girl Scout® Lemonades | | | Free of lactose. | |
| Girl Scout® Peanut Butter Patties | | | Free of lactose. | |
| Girl Scout® Samoas® | 52¼ | | Piece (14.5g); 758g in total. | +43½ |
| Girl Scout® Shortbread® | 18½ | | Piece (11.34g); 210g in total. | +15½ |
| Girl Scout® Thin Mints | 32½ | | Piece (8g); 260g in total. | +27 |
| Halvah | | | Free of lactose. | |
| Lebkuchen (German ginger bread) | | | Nearly free of lactose | |
| Little Debbie® Coffee Cake, Apple Streusel | | | Free of lactose. | |
| Little Debbie® Fudge Brownies with Walnuts | | | Free of lactose. | |
| Long John or Bismarck, glazed, cream or custard filled & nuts | 2¼ | | Piece (105g); 236g in total. | +2 |
| Molasses cookies, store bought | | | Free of lactose. | |
| Muffins, banana | 1¼ | | Piece (113g); 141g in total. | +1 |

| Sweet pastries | LACTOSE | | Standard amount | |
|---|---|---|---|---|
| Muffins, blueberry, store bought | 1¼ | | Piece (113g); 141g in total. | +1 |
| Muffins, carrot, homemade, with nuts | 1¼ | | Piece (113g); 141g in total. | +1 |
| Muffins, oat bran or oatmeal, store bought | 1¼ | | Piece (113g); 141g in total. | +1 |
| Muffins, pumpkin, store bought | 1¼ | | Piece (113g); 141g in total. | +1 |
| Murray® Sugar Free Oatmeal Cookies | | | Free of lactose. | |
| Murray® Sugar Free Shortbread | | | Free of lactose. | |
| Nabisco® 100 Calorie Packs, Honey Maid Cinnamon Roll | | | Free of lactose. | |
| Nilla Wafers® (Nabisco®) | 32½ | | Piece (3.75g); 122g in total. | +27 |
| Nutter Butter® Cookies (Nabisco®) | | | Free of lactose. | |
| Oatmeal cookies, store bought | 45¾ | | Piece (13g); 595g in total. | +38 |
| Oreo® Brownie Cookies (Nabisco®) | | | Nearly free of lactose | |
| Oreo® Cookies (Nabisco®) | | | Free of lactose. | |
| Oreo® Cookies, Sugar Free (Nabisco®) | | | Nearly free of lactose | |
| Pancake, buckwheat, from mix, add water only | | | Free of lactose. | |
| Pancake, whole wheat, home-made | 2½ | | Piece (44g); 110g in total. | +2 |
| Peach pie, bottom crust only | | | Free of lactose. | |

| Sweet pastries | LACTOSE | Standard amount | |
|---|---|---|---|
| Pepperidge Farm® Sweet & Simple, Soft Sugar Cookies | ☺ | Nearly free of lactose | |
| Pepperidge Farm® Turnover, Apple | 9 | Piece (89g); 801g in total. | +7½ |
| Pillsbury® Big White Chunk Macadamia Nut Cookies | 6¾ | Piece (38g); 257g in total. | +5½ |
| Pillsbury® Cinnamon Roll with Icing, all flavors | 9 | Piece (44g); 396g in total. | +7½ |
| Popcorn, store bought (prepopped), "buttered" | 36¾ | Portion (30g); 1103g in total. | +30¾ |
| Rhubarb pie, bottom crust only | ☺ | Free of lactose. | |
| Sandwich cookies, vanilla | 9 | Piece (15g); 135g in total. | +7½ |
| Sticky bun | 8¾ | Piece (71g); 621g in total. | +7¼ |
| Strawberry pie, bottom crust only | ☺ | Free of lactose. | |
| Sugar cookies, iced, store bought | ☺ | Nearly free of lactose | |
| Sweet potato bread | ☺ | Nearly free of lactose | |
| Tiramisu | 2½ | Portion (55g); 138g in total. | +2 |
| Twix® | 2 | Piece (51g); 102g in total. | +1¾ |
| Waffles, bran | ¾ | Piece (95g); 71g in total. | +¾ |
| Waffles, whole wheat, from mix, add milk, fat and egg | 1 | Piece (95g); 95g in total. | +¾ |
| Windmill cookies | ☺ | Free of lactose. | |

# 3.4.7 Sweets

| Sweets | LACTOSE | | Standard amount | ⊕ |
|---|---|---|---|---|
| 3 Musketeers® | 1¾ | | Piece (60.4g); 106g in total. | +1½ |
| After Eight® Thin Chocolate Mints | 10¼ | | Piece (8g); 82g in total. | +8½ |
| Almond paste (Marzipan) | | ☺ | Free of lactose. | |
| Almonds, honey roasted | | ☺ | Free of lactose. | |
| Breath mint, regular | | ☺ | Free of lactose. | |
| Breath mint, sugar free | | ☺ | Free of lactose. | |
| Brown sugar | | ☺ | Free of lactose. | |
| Buttermels® (Switzer's®) | 8 | | Piece (6.9g); 55g in total. | +6½ |
| Candy necklace | | ☺ | Free of lactose. | |
| Chewing gum | | ☺ | Free of lactose. | |
| Chewing gum, sugar free | | ☺ | Free of lactose. | |
| Chocolate truffles | 2½ | | Piece (16.2g); 41g in total. | +2 |
| Classic Fruit Chocolates (Liberty Orchards®) | 56½ | | Piece (15g); 848g in total. | +47 |
| Coconut Bars, nuts | 45¼ | | Piece (42g); 1901g in total. | +37¾ |
| Dark chocolate Bar 45%-59% cacao | 1¼ | | 135g Bar (125g); 156g in total. | +1 |

| Sweets | LACTOSE | Standard amount | |
|---|---|---|---|
| Dark chocolate Bar 60%-69% cacao | 7½ | 135g Bar (125g); 938g in total. | +6¼ |
| Dark chocolate Bar 70%-85% cacao | | 😊 Free of lactose. | |
| Dark chocolate Bar, sugar free | 26¾ | Piece (12g); 321g in total. | +22¼ |
| Dark Fruit Chocolates (Liberty Orchards®) | 56½ | Piece (15g); 848g in total. | +47 |
| Dark Fruit Chocolates, Sugar Free (Liberty Orchards®) | 37¾ | Piece (17g); 642g in total. | +31¼ |
| Fifty 50® Sugar Free Low Glycemic Butterscotch Hard Candy | | 😊 Free of lactose. | |
| French Burnt Peanuts | | 😊 Free of lactose. | |
| Gelatin (jello) powder, flavored, sugar free | | 😊 Free of lactose. | |
| Gelatin (jello) powder, plain | | 😊 Free of lactose. | |
| Gum drops | | 😊 Free of lactose. | |
| Gum drops, sugar free | | 😊 Free of lactose. | |
| Gummi bears | | 😊 Free of lactose. | |
| Gummi bears, sugar free | | 😊 Free of lactose. | |
| Gummi dinosaurs | | 😊 Free of lactose. | |
| Gummi dinosaurs, sugar free | | 😊 Free of lactose. | |
| Gummi worms | | 😊 Free of lactose. | |

| Sweets | LACTOSE | | Standard amount | |
|---|---|---|---|---|
| Marshmallow | | 🙂 | Free of lactose. | |
| Mentos® | | 🙂 | Free of lactose. | |
| Milk chocolate Bar, cereal | ½ | | 135g Bar (125g); 63g in total. | +½ |
| Milk chocolate Bar, cereal, sugar free | 7½ | | Piece (12g); 90g in total. | +6¼ |
| Milk chocolate Bar, sugar free | 3¼ | | Piece (12g); 39g in total. | +2½ |
| Milk Chocolate covered raisins | 2¾ | | Hand (30g); 83g in total. | +2¼ |
| Milk Maid® Caramels (Brach's®) | ½ | | Piece (40g); 20g in total. | +¼ |
| Molasses, dark | | 🙂 | Free of lactose. | |
| Nestle® Nesquik®, chocolate flavors, unprepared dry | | | Glass (240g); Avoid consumption!! | 0.19 |
| Nougat | | 🙂 | Free of lactose. | |
| Pecan praline | 3½ | | Piece (55g); 193g in total. | +2¾ |
| Riesen® | 12¾ | | Piece (9g); 115g in total. | +10½ |
| Smarties® | | 🙂 | Free of lactose. | |
| Snickers® | 1½ | | Piece (58.7g); 88g in total. | +1¼ |
| Snickers®, Almond | 1¾ | | Piece (49.9g); 87g in total. | +1½ |
| Splenda® | | 🙂 | Free of lactose. | |

| Sweets | LACTOSE | Standard amount | |
|---|---|---|---|
| Starburst®, Original | 😊 | Free of lactose. | |
| Suckers®, sugar free | 😊 | Free of lactose. | |
| Sugar, white granulated | 😊 | Free of lactose. | |
| Taffy | 😊 | Free of lactose. | |
| Tic Tacs® | 😊 | Free of lactose. | |
| Toblerone® Swiss Dark Chocolate with Honey & Almond Nougat | 7¼ | Piece (25g); 181g in total. | +6 |
| Toblerone® Swiss Milk Chocolate with Honey & Almond Nougat | 1½ | Piece (25g); 38g in total. | +1¼ |
| Toblerone® Swiss White Confection with Honey & Almond Nougat | 1 | Piece (25g); 25g in total. | +1 |
| Toffee | 40¾ | Piece (7g); 285g in total. | +34 |
| Toffifay® | 7½ | Piece (8.2g); 62g in total. | +6¼ |
| Tootsie Pops® | 😊 | Free of lactose. | |
| Werther's® Original Caramel Coffee Hard Candies | 17¾ | Piece (4g); 71g in total. | +14¾ |
| White chocolate Bar | 2½ | Piece (12g); 30g in total. | +2 |
| Wild 'n Fruity Gummi Bears (Brach's®) | 😊 | Free of lactose. | |
| Zsweet® | 😊 | Free of lactose. | |

# 3.5 Warm dishes

## 3.5.1 Meals

| Meals | LACTOSE | | Standard amount | 🔵 |
|---|---|---|---|---|
| Arby's® macaroni and cheese | 21½ | | Portion (217g); 4666g in total. | +18 |
| Asian noodle bowl, vegetables only | | 😊 | Free of lactose. | |
| Baby food, Gerber Graduates® Organic Pasta Pick-Ups Three Cheese Ravioli | 1 | | Portion (170g); 170g in total. | +¾ |
| Beef with noodles soup, condensed | | 😊 | Free of lactose. | |
| Boston Market® macaroni and cheese | ½ | | Portion (243g); 122g in total. | +½ |
| Butternut squash soup | 13½ | | Portion (245g); 3308g in total. | +11¼ |
| Calzone, cheese | 12¼ | | Piece (168g); 2058g in total. | +10¼ |
| Casserole (hot dish), pasta with turkey, gravy base, vegetables other than dark green, cheese | 3¾ | | Portion (228g); 855g in total. | +3 |
| Casserole (hot dish), rice with beef, tomato base, vegetables other than dark green, cheese | 9¾ | | Portion (244g); 2379g in total. | +8¼ |
| Chicken and dumplings soup, condensed | 7¼ | | Portion (126g); 914g in total. | +6 |
| Chicken noodle soup with vegetables, ready-to-serve can | | 😊 | Free of lactose. | |
| Chicken wonton soup, prepared from condensed can | | 😊 | Free of lactose. | |
| Chili with beans, beef, canned | | 😊 | Free of lactose. | |

| Meals | LACTOSE | | Standard amount | |
|---|---|---|---|---|
| Chop suey, chicken, no noodles | | 😊 | Free of lactose. | |
| Chop suey, tofu, no noodles | | 😊 | Free of lactose. | |
| Cream of asparagus soup, prepared from condensed can | 6½ | 🥄 | Tbsp. (15g); 98g in total. | +5½ |
| Cream of broccoli soup, condensed | 5 | 🍲 | Portion (126g); 630g in total. | +4¼ |
| Cream of celery soup, homemade | ½ | 🍲 | Portion (245g); 123g in total. | +½ |
| Cream of chicken soup, condensed | 6½ | 🍲 | Portion (126g); 819g in total. | +5½ |
| Cream of mushroom soup, prepared from condensed can | 1½ | 🍲 | Portion (245g); 368g in total. | +1¼ |
| Cream of potato soup mix, dry | 3¼ | 🍲 | Portion (23g); 75g in total. | +2¾ |
| Cream of spinach soup mix, dry | | 😊 | Free of lactose. | |
| Dairy Queen® Foot Long Hot Dog | | 😊 | Free of lactose. | |
| Fettuccini Alfredo®, no meat, vegetables except dark green | ¾ | 🍲 | Portion (200g); 150g in total. | +¾ |
| Fettuccini Alfredo®, no meat, carrots or dark green vegetables | 5 | 🍲 | Portion (200g); 1000g in total. | +4 |
| Fruit sauce, jelly-based | | 😊 | Free of lactose. | |
| German style potato salad, with bacon and vinegar dressing | | 😊 | Free of lactose. | |
| Green pea soup, prepared from condensed can | | 😊 | Free of lactose. | |
| Hardee's® Loaded Omelet Biscuit | 12 | 🍰 | Piece (158g); 1896g in total. | +10 |

| Meals | LACTOSE | | Standard amount | |
|---|---|---|---|---|
| Lasagna, homemade, beef | 2 | | Portion (140g); 280g in total. | +1¾ |
| Lasagna, homemade, cheese, no vegetables | 1¼ | | Portion (140g); 175g in total. | +1 |
| Lasagna, homemade, spinach, no meat | 8½ | | Portion (140g); 1190g in total. | +7 |
| Lentil soup, condensed | | ☺ | Nearly free of lactose | |
| Lyonnaise (potatoes and onions) | | ☺ | Free of lactose. | |
| Macaroni or pasta salad, with meat, egg, mayo dressing | | ☺ | Free of lactose. | |
| Meat ravioli, with tomato sauce | | ☺ | Nearly free of lactose | |
| Minestrone soup, condensed | | ☺ | Free of lactose. | |
| Minestrone soup, homemade | | ☺ | Free of lactose. | |
| Noodle soup mix, dry | | ☺ | Free of lactose. | |
| Omelet, made with bacon | 34¾ | | Portion (110g); 3823g in total. | +29 |
| Omelet, made with sausage, potatoes, onions, cheese | 52¼ | | Portion (110g); 5748g in total. | +43½ |
| Pad Thai, without meat | | ☺ | Free of lactose. | |
| Paella | | ☺ | Free of lactose. | |
| Panda Express® Orange Chicken | 6½ | | Portion (140g); 910g in total. | +5¼ |
| Pasta salad with vegetables, Italian dressing | | ☺ | Nearly free of lactose | |

| Meals | LACTOSE | | Standard amount | |
|---|---|---|---|---|
| Pho soup (Vietnamese noodle soup) | | 😊 | Free of lactose. | |
| Pizza Hut® cheese bread stick | 61½ | 🍰 | Piece (56g); 3444g in total. | +51¼ |
| Pizza Hut® Pepperoni Lover's pizza, stuffed crust | 30 | 🥘 | Portion (140g); 4200g in total. | +25 |
| Pizza Hut® Personal Pan, supreme | 16¾ | 🍰 | Piece (256g); 4288g in total. | +14 |
| Pizza, homemade or restaurant, cheese, thin crust | 12¼ | 🍰 | Piece (209g); 2560g in total. | +10¼ |
| Potato salad, with egg, mayo dressing | | 😊 | Free of lactose. | |
| Potato soup with broccoli and cheese | 29¾ | 🥘 | Portion (245g); 7289g in total. | +24¾ |
| Ratatouille | | 😊 | Nearly free of lactose | |
| Red beans and rice soup mix, dry | | 😊 | Free of lactose. | |
| Scrambled egg, made with bacon | 2¼ | 🥘 | Portion (110g); 248g in total. | +1¾ |
| Sesame chicken | | 😊 | Free of lactose. | |
| Soup base | | 😊 | Free of lactose. | |
| Spaghetti, with carbonara sauce | 13½ | 🥘 | Portion (201g); 2714g in total. | +11¼ |
| Spinach ravioli, with tomato sauce | 5½ | 🥘 | Portion (250g); 1375g in total. | +4½ |
| Spring roll | | 😊 | Free of lactose. | |
| Squash or pumpkin ravioli, with cream sauce | ½ | 🥘 | Portion (250g); 125g in total. | +½ |

| Meals | LACTOSE | | Standard amount | |
|-------|---------|---|----------------|---|
| Stewed green peas with sofrito | | 😊 | Free of lactose. | |
| Sushi, with fish | | 😊 | Free of lactose. | |
| Sushi, with fish and vegetables in seaweed | | 😊 | Free of lactose. | |
| Sushi, with vegetables in seaweed | | 😊 | Free of lactose. | |
| Swedish Meatballs | 1½ | 🍲 | Portion (140g); 210g in total. | +1¼ |
| Sweet and sour chicken | | 😊 | Free of lactose. | |
| Taco Bell® 7-Layer Burrito | 25½ | 🍲 | Portion (140g); 3570g in total. | +21¼ |
| Taco Bell® Crunchwrap Supreme | 4¼ | 🍰 | Piece (245g); 1041g in total. | +3½ |
| Taco Bell® Mexican Pizza | 13¾ | 🍰 | Piece (213g); 2929g in total. | +11½ |
| Taco Bell® Nachos Supreme | 6¼ | 🍲 | Portion (140g); 875g in total. | +5¼ |
| Taco, soft corn shell, with beans, cheese | | 😊 | Nearly free of lactose | +77½ |
| Tomato relish | | 😊 | Free of lactose. | |
| Tomato soup mix, dry | ¼ | 🍲 | Portion (34.66g); 9g in total. | 0.24 |
| Vegetable soup, condensed | | 😊 | Free of lactose. | |
| Vichyssoise | ¾ | 🍲 | Portion (245g); 184g in total. | +½ |
| White bean stew with sofrito | | 😊 | Free of lactose. | |

## 3.5.2   Meat and fish

| Meat and fish | LACTOSE | Standard amount | |
|---|---|---|---|
| Beef bacon (kosher) | ☺ | Free of lactose. | |
| Beef steak, chuck, visible fat eaten | ☺ | Free of lactose. | |
| Bockwurst | ☺ | Free of lactose. | |
| Boston Market® 1/4 white rotisserie chicken, with skin | ☺ | Free of lactose. | |
| Boston Market® roasted turkey breast | ☺ | Free of lactose. | |
| Bratwurst | ☺ | Free of lactose. | |
| Bratwurst, beef | ☺ | Free of lactose. | |
| Bratwurst, light (reduced fat) | ☺ | Free of lactose. | |
| Bratwurst, made with beer | ☺ | Free of lactose. | |
| Bratwurst, made with beer, cheese-filled | ☺ | Nearly free of lactose | |
| Bratwurst, turkey | ☺ | Free of lactose. | |
| Braunschweiger | ☺ | Free of lactose. | |
| Caviar | ☺ | Free of lactose. | |
| Chicken fricassee with gravy, American style | ☺ | Free of lactose. | |
| Clams, stuffed with mushroom, onions, and bread | 24½ | Portion (140g); 3430g in total. | +20½ |

| Meat and fish | LACTOSE | | Standard amount | |
|---|---|---|---|---|
| Clams, stuffed with mushroom, onions, and bread | 24½ | | Portion (140g); 3430g in total. | +20½ |
| Fish croquette | 2¼ | | Portion (85g); 191g in total. | +1¾ |
| Fish sticks, patties, or nuggets, breaded, regular | | | Free of lactose. | |
| Fish with breading | | | Free of lactose. | |
| Gorton's® Battered Fish Fillets - Lemon Pepper | | | Free of lactose. | |
| Gorton's® Popcorn Shrimp, Original | | | Free of lactose. | |
| Goulash, with beef, noodles or macaroni, tomato base | | | Free of lactose. | |
| Herring, pickled | | | Free of lactose. | |
| Herring, pickled | | | Free of lactose. | |
| Liver pudding | | | Free of lactose. | |
| Mrs. Paul's® Calamari Rings | | | Nearly free of lactose | |
| Pickled beef | | | Free of lactose. | |
| Pork cutlet (sirloin cutlet), visible fat eaten | | | Free of lactose. | |
| Ribs, beef, spare, visible fat eaten | | | Free of lactose. | |
| Salami, beer or beerwurst, beef | | | Free of lactose. | |
| Salmon, red (sockeye), smoked | | | Free of lactose. | |

| Meat and fish | LACTOSE | Standard amount | |
|---|---|---|---|
| Sauerbraten | 😊 | Free of lactose. | |
| Scallops | 😊 | Free of lactose. | |
| Sea Pak® Seasoned Shrimp, Roasted Garlic | 😊 | Free of lactose. | |
| Sea Pak® Shrimp Scampi in Italian Parmesan Sauce | 😊 | Nearly free of lactose | |
| Spiced ham loaf (e.g. Spam), canned | 😊 | Free of lactose. | |
| Tuna, canned, light, oil pack, not drained | 😊 | Free of lactose. | |
| Venison or deer, stewed | 😊 | Free of lactose. | |

## 3.5.3 Lactose hideouts

| Lactose hideouts | LACTOSE | Standard amount | |
|---|---|---|---|
| Casserole (hot dish), chicken with pasta, cream or white sauce, with cheese | ½ | Portion (238g); 119g in total. | |
| Chicken cake or patty | 1½ | Portion (85g); 128g in total. | 3¼ |
| Chicken with cheese sauce, vegetables other than dark green | ½ | Portion (216g); 108g in total. | |
| Creamed chicken | ½ | Portion (241g); 121g in total. | |
| Fish croquette | 1¾ | Portion (85g); 149g in total. | 1¾ |
| Fish or seafood with cream or white sauce | 1½ | Portion (181g); 272g in total. | |
| Ham croquette | 2¼ | Portion (85g); 191g in total. | |
| Loaf cold cut, spiced | 2¼ | Portion (55g); 124g in total. | |
| Meatloaf, pork | 2¼ | Portion (85g); 191g in total. | |
| Meatloaf, tuna | 5½ | Portion (85g); 468g in total. | |
| Soufflé, meat | 1¼ | Portion (110g); 138g in total. | 1¾ |
| Swedish Meatballs | 1½ | Portion (140g); 210g in total. | 9 |

# 3.5.4 Side dishes

| Side dishes | LACTOSE | | Standard amount | |
|---|---|---|---|---|
| Au gratin potato, prepared from fresh | 1 | | Portion (140g); 140g in total. | +¾ |
| Basmati rice, cooked in unsalted water | | | Free of lactose. | |
| Boston Market® sweet corn | | | Free of lactose. | |
| Bulgur, home cooked | | | Free of lactose. | |
| Cheese gnocchi | 3½ | | Portion (70g); 245g in total. | +2¾ |
| Cornbread, from mix | 4¾ | | Portion (55g); 261g in total. | +3¾ |
| Cornbread, homemade | 2¾ | | Portion (55g); 151g in total. | +2¼ |
| Couscous, cooked | | | Free of lactose. | |
| Falafel | | | Free of lactose. | |
| Fettuccini noodles, whole wheat, cooked in unsalted water | | | Free of lactose. | |
| Garbanzo beans (chickpeas), canned, drained | | | Free of lactose. | |
| Green peas, raw | | | Free of lactose. | |
| Kidney beans, cooked from dried | | | Free of lactose. | |
| Lentils, cooked from dried | | | Free of lactose. | |
| Plain dumplings for stew, biscuit type | 1¾ | | Portion (55g); 96g in total. | +1½ |

| Side dishes | LACTOSE | Standard amount | |
|---|---|---|---|
| Polenta | ½ | Portion (240g); 120g in total. | +½ |
| Potato dumpling (Kartoffelkloesse) | 45½ | Portion (140g); 6370g in total. | +37¾ |
| Potato gnocchi | | Free of lactose. | |
| Potato pancakes | | Free of lactose. | |
| Potato, boiled, with skin | | Free of lactose. | |
| Potato, boiled, without skin | | Free of lactose. | |
| Quinoa, cooked | | Free of lactose. | |
| Rice noodles, fried | | Free of lactose. | |
| Snow peas (edible pea pods), cooked from fresh | | Free of lactose. | |
| Spaetzle (spatzen) | 5¼ | Portion (140g); 735g in total. | +4¼ |

# 3.6 Fast food chains

## 3.6.1 Burger King®

| Burger King® | LACTOSE | | Standard amount | ⊕ |
|---|---|---|---|---|
| Bacon EGG® and Cheese BK Muffin® | 11½ | | Piece (131g); 1507g in total. | +9½ |
| Barbecue sauce | | ☺ | Free of lactose. | |
| BBQ roasted jalapeno sauce | | ☺ | Free of lactose. | |
| BK Big Fish® | | ☺ | Free of lactose. | |
| BK Fresh Apple Slices | | ☺ | Free of lactose. | |
| BLT Salad® with TenderCrisp chicken (no dressing or croutons) | 79¼ | | Portion (140g); 11095g in total. | +66 |
| Caesar Salad (no dressing or croutons) | 26½ | | Portion (100g); 2650g in total. | +22 |
| Cheeseburger | 11½ | | Piece (121g); 1392g in total. | +9½ |
| French fries | | ☺ | Free of lactose. | |
| Hamburger | | ☺ | Free of lactose. | |
| Ken's® Apple Cider Vinaigrette salad dressing | | ☺ | Nearly free of lactose | |
| Onion rings | | ☺ | Free of lactose. | |
| Original Chicken Crisp® Sandwich | | ☺ | Free of lactose. | |

| Burger King® | LACTOSE | | Standard amount | |
|---|---|---|---|---|
| Pancakes and syrup | ½ | | Piece (187g); 94g in total. | +½ |
| Picante taco sauce | | | Free of lactose. | |
| Ranch Crispy Chicken Wrap | 5 | | Piece (137g); 685g in total. | +4¼ |
| Shake, chocolate | | | Portion (231g); Avoid consumption!! | 0.15 |
| Shake, strawberry | | | Portion (229g); Avoid consumption!! | 0.15 |
| Shake, vanilla or other | | | Portion (238g); Avoid consumption!! | 0.14 |
| Sundaes®, caramel | ¼ | | Portion (141g); 35g in total. | +¼ |
| Sundaes®, chocolate fudge | ¼ | | Portion (141g); 35g in total. | +¼ |
| Sundaes®, mini M & M® | ¼ | | Portion (204g); 51g in total. | 0.24 |
| Sundaes®, Oreo® | ¼ | | Portion (204g); 51g in total. | +¼ |
| Sundaes®, strawberry | ¼ | | Portion (141g); 35g in total. | +¼ |
| Sweet and sour sauce | | | Free of lactose. | |
| TenderCrisp® Chicken Sandwich | | | Free of lactose. | |
| Whopper® with cheese | 5¾ | | Piece (315g); 1811g in total. | +4¾ |
| Zesty onion ring sauce | | | Nearly free of lactose | |

# 3.6.2 KFC®

| KFC® | LACTOSE | Standard amount | |
|---|---|---|---|
| Caesar salad dressing | 4¾ | Portion (30g); 143g in total. | +3¾ |
| Chicken breast, spicy crispy | | Free of lactose. | |
| Chicken Littles with sauce | | Free of lactose. | |
| Cole slaw | | Free of lactose. | |
| Creamy buffalo sauce | 6 | Portion (29.4g); 176g in total. | +5 |
| Crispy Chicken Caesar Salad | | Nearly free of lactose | |
| Crispy Twister without sauce | | Free of lactose. | |
| Crispy Twister® with sauce | | Free of lactose. | |
| Extra Crispy Tenders | | Free of lactose. | |
| Honey BBQ sauce | | Free of lactose. | |
| Hot wings | | Free of lactose. | |
| House side salad | | Free of lactose. | |
| Mashed potatoes with gravy | ½ | Portion (140g); 70g in total. | +½ |
| Sweet and sour sauce | | Free of lactose. | |
| Sweet corn | | Free of lactose. | |

## 3.6.3 McDonald's®

| McDonald's® | LACTOSE | | Standard amount | |
|---|---|---|---|---|
| McDonald's® apple slices | | ☺ | Free of lactose. | |
| McDonald's® Barbecue sauce | | ☺ | Free of lactose. | |
| McDonald's® Big Mac® | 9¾ | 🍰 | Piece (215g); 2096g in total. | +8¼ |
| McDonald's® caramel sundae® | ¼ | 🥄 | Portion (182g); 46g in total. | +¼ |
| McDonald's® Cheeseburger | 9¾ | 🍰 | Piece (114g); 1112g in total. | +8¼ |
| McDonald's® Chicken McNuggets® | | ☺ | Free of lactose. | |
| McDonald's® chocolate chip cookies | | ☺ | Free of lactose. | |
| McDonald's® chocolate milk | ¼ | ☕ | Cup (150g); 38 mL in total. | +¼ |
| McDonald's® Crispy Chicken Snack Wrap with ranch sauce | 62 | 🍰 | Piece (118g); 7316g in total. | +51½ |
| McDonald's® Double Cheeseburger | 4¾ | 🍰 | Piece (165g); 784g in total. | +4 |
| McDonald's® Filet-O-Fish® | 19¾ | 🍰 | Piece (142g); 2805g in total. | +16½ |
| McDonald's® French fries | | ☺ | Free of lactose. | |
| McDonald's® Hamburger | | ☺ | Free of lactose. | |
| McDonald's® hot fudge sundae® | ¼ | 🥄 | Portion (179g); 45g in total. | +¼ |
| McDonald's® hot mustard sauce | | ☺ | Nearly free of lactose | |

| McDonald's® | LACTOSE | | Standard amount | |
|---|---|---|---|---|
| McDonald's® M & M McFlurry® | | | Portion (228g); Avoid consumption!! | 0.19 |
| McDonald's® McCafe shakes, chocolate flavors | ¼ | | Portion (210g); 53g in total. | +¼ |
| McDonald's® McCafe shakes, vanilla or other flavors | ¼ | | Portion (206g); 52g in total. | +¼ |
| McDonald's® McChicken® | | ☺ | Free of lactose. | |
| McDonald's® McDouble® | 9¾ | | Piece (151g); 1472g in total. | +8¼ |
| McDonald's® McRib® | | ☺ | Free of lactose. | |
| McDonald's® Newman's Own® Creamy Caesar salad dressing | 18¼ | | Portion (30g); 548g in total. | +15¼ |
| McDonald's® Newman's Own® Low Fat Balsamic Vinaigrette salad dressing | | ☺ | Free of lactose. | |
| McDonald's® orange juice | | ☺ | Free of lactose. | |
| McDonald's® Quarter Pounder | | ☺ | Free of lactose. | |
| McDonald's® Sausage & EGG® McMuffin® | 9¾ | | Piece (164g); 1599g in total. | +8¼ |
| McDonald's® side salad | | ☺ | Free of lactose. | |
| McDonald's® smoothies, all flavors | 2¼ | | Glass (240g); 540 mL in total. | +1¾ |
| McDonald's® Southwestern chipotle Barbecue sauce | | ☺ | Free of lactose. | |
| McDonald's® sweet and sour sauce | | ☺ | Free of lactose. | |

## 3.6.4 Subway®

| Subway® | LACTOSE | | Standard amount | |
|---|---|---|---|---|
| 9-grain Wheat bread | | ☺ | Free of lactose. | |
| American cheese | 4½ | 🍽 | Portion (30g); 135g in total. | +3¾ |
| bacon | | ☺ | Free of lactose. | |
| Cheddar cheese | 43¼ | 🍽 | Portion (30g); 1298g in total. | +36 |
| Chipotle southwest salad dressing | 7¼ | 🍽 | Portion (30g); 218g in total. | +6 |
| Chocolate chip cookie | 6¾ | 🍰 | Piece (45g); 304g in total. | +5½ |
| Chocolate chunk cookie | 6¾ | 🍰 | Piece (45g); 304g in total. | +5½ |
| Ham Sandwich with Veggies, no mayo | 12½ | 🍰 | Piece (219g); 2738g in total. | +10½ |
| Honey mustard salad dressing | | ☺ | Free of lactose. | |
| Honey Oat bread | ¾ | 🍰 | Piece (89g); 67g in total. | +½ |
| Italian BMT® Sandwich with Veggies, no mayo | 12½ | 🍰 | Piece (226g); 2825g in total. | +10½ |
| M & M® cookie | 6¾ | 🍰 | Piece (45g); 304g in total. | +5½ |
| Mustard | | ☺ | Free of lactose. | |
| Oven Roasted Chicken Sandwich with Veggies, no mayo | 12½ | 🍰 | Piece (233g); 2913g in total. | +10½ |
| Parmesan Oregano bread | | ☺ | Nearly free of lactose | |

| Subway® | LACTOSE | | Standard amount | |
|---|---|---|---|---|
| Ranch salad dressing | | ☺ | Nearly free of lactose | |
| Roast Beef Sandwich with Veggies, no mayo | 12½ | 🍰 | Piece (233g); 2913g in total. | +10½ |
| Spicy Italian Sandwich with Veggies, no meat | 12½ | 🍰 | Piece (222g); 2775g in total. | +10½ |
| Steak & Cheese Sandwich with Veggies, no mayo | | ☺ | Nearly free of lactose | |
| Sweet Onion Chicken Teriyaki Sandwich with Veggies, no mayo | 12½ | 🍰 | Piece (276g); 3450g in total. | +10½ |
| Sweet onion salad dressing | | ☺ | Free of lactose. | |
| Tuna Sandwich with Veggies, no mayo | 12½ | 🍰 | Piece (233g); 2913g in total. | +10½ |
| Turkey Breast & Ham Sandwich with Veggies, no mayo | 12½ | 🍰 | Piece (219g); 2738g in total. | +10½ |
| Turkey Breast Sandwich with Veggies, no mayo | 12½ | 🍰 | Piece (219g); 2738g in total. | +10½ |
| Veggie Delite Salad, no dressing | 34¼ | 🥗 | Portion (100g); 3425g in total. | +28½ |
| Veggie Delite Sandwich, no mayo | 12½ | 🍰 | Piece (162g); 2025g in total. | +10½ |
| Vinegar | | ☺ | Free of lactose. | |
| White chip macadamia nut cookie | 6¾ | 🍰 | Piece (45g); 304g in total. | +5½ |
| Wrap bread | | ☺ | Free of lactose. | |

## 3.6.5  Taco Bell®

| Taco Bell® | LACTOSE | | Standard amount | ☕ |
|---|---|---|---|---|
| Chalupas Supreme® with beef, beans, cheese | 49¾ | | Portion (140g); 6965g in total. | +41½ |
| Taco Bell® Beef Enchirito | 69 | | Portion (140g); 9660g in total. | +57½ |
| Taco Bell® Caramel Apple Empanada | 10½ | | Portion (125g); 1313g in total. | +8¾ |
| Taco Bell® Cheesy Fiesta Potatos | 4 | | Portion (140g); 560g in total. | +3¼ |
| Taco Bell® cheesy gordita crunch | 15 | | Portion (140g); 2100g in total. | +12½ |
| Taco Bell® Cinnamon Twists | | ☺ | Free of lactose. | |
| Taco Bell® Combo Burrito | | ☺ | Nearly free of lactose | |
| Taco Bell® Double Decker Taco Supreme®, beef | 61 | | Portion (140g); 8540g in total. | +51 |
| Taco Bell® Pintos 'n Cheese | 17 | | Portion (130g); 2210g in total. | +14 |

# 3.6.6 Wendy's®

| Wendy's® | LACTOSE | | Standard amount | |
|---|---|---|---|---|
| Strawberry Shake | ¼ | | Glass (200g); 50 mL in total. | +¼ |
| Wendys' chili cheese fries | 2½ | | Portion (140g); 350g in total. | +2¼ |
| Wendy's® Baconator® | 13 | | Portion (140g); 1820g in total. | +10¾ |
| Wendy's® Baked Potato, with sour cream and chives | | | Nearly free of lactose | |
| Wendy's® Caesar side salad | 9 | | Portion (100g); 900g in total. | +7½ |
| Wendy's® Chicken Nuggets | | | Free of lactose. | |
| Wendy's® French fries | | | Free of lactose. | |
| Wendy's® Frosty Float® | ¼ | | Portion (192g); 48g in total. | +¼ |
| Wendy's® Jr. Bacon Cheeseburger | 13¾ | | Portion (140g); 1925g in total. | +11½ |
| Wendy's® Jr. Cheeseburger Deluxe | 14 | | Portion (140g); 1960g in total. | +11¾ |
| Wendy's® side salad | | | Free of lactose. | |
| Wendy's® Spicy Chicken Go Wrap | 31½ | | Portion (140g); 4410g in total. | +26¼ |
| Wendy's® Spicy Chicken Sandwich | | | Free of lactose. | |

# 3.7 Fruits and vegetables

## 3.7.1 Fruit

| Fruit | LACTOSE | Standard amount | |
|---|---|---|---|
| Applesauce, canned, sweetened | ☺ | Free of lactose. | |
| Applesauce, canned, unsweetened | ☺ | Free of lactose. | |
| Apricot, dried, cooked, sweetened | ☺ | Free of lactose. | |
| Apricot, dried, uncooked | ☺ | Free of lactose. | |
| Apricot, fresh | ☺ | Free of lactose. | |
| Banana, chips | ☺ | Free of lactose. | |
| Banana, fresh | ☺ | Free of lactose. | |
| Blackberries, fresh | ☺ | Free of lactose. | |
| Blueberries, fresh | ☺ | Free of lactose. | |
| Boysenberries, fresh | ☺ | Free of lactose. | |
| Cantaloupe, fresh | ☺ | Free of lactose. | |
| Carambola (starfruit), fresh | ☺ | Free of lactose. | |
| Clementine, fresh | ☺ | Free of lactose. | |

| Fruit | LACTOSE | Standard amount |
|---|---|---|
| Cranberries, dried (Craisins®) | 😊 | Free of lactose. |
| Cranberries, fresh | 😊 | Free of lactose. |
| Currants, fresh, black | 😊 | Free of lactose. |
| Currants, fresh, red and white | 😊 | Free of lactose. |
| Dates | 😊 | Free of lactose. |
| Elderberries, fresh | 😊 | Free of lactose. |
| Figs, dried, cooked, sweetened | 😊 | Free of lactose. |
| Figs, fresh | 😊 | Free of lactose. |
| Gooseberries, fresh | 😊 | Free of lactose. |
| Grapefruit, fresh, pink or red | 😊 | Free of lactose. |
| Grapes, fresh | 😊 | Free of lactose. |
| Guava (guayaba), fresh, common | 😊 | Free of lactose. |
| Honeydew | 😊 | Free of lactose. |
| Jackfruit, fresh | 😊 | Free of lactose. |
| Kiwi fruit, gold | 😊 | Free of lactose. |
| Kiwi fruit, green | 😊 | Free of lactose. |

| Fruit | LACTOSE | Standard amount |
|---|---|---|
| Lemon, fresh | ☺ | Free of lactose. |
| Lime, fresh | ☺ | Free of lactose. |
| Loganberries, fresh | ☺ | Free of lactose. |
| Lowbush cranberries (lingonberries) | ☺ | Free of lactose. |
| Lychees (litchis), fresh | ☺ | Free of lactose. |
| Lycium (wolf or goji berries) | ☺ | Free of lactose. |
| Mandarin orange, fresh | ☺ | Free of lactose. |
| Mango, fresh | ☺ | Free of lactose. |
| Mangosteen, fresh | ☺ | Free of lactose. |
| Mulberries | ☺ | Free of lactose. |
| Muskmelon | ☺ | Free of lactose. |
| Nectarine, fresh | ☺ | Free of lactose. |
| Orange, fresh | ☺ | Free of lactose. |
| Papaya, fresh | ☺ | Free of lactose. |
| Passion fruit (maracuya), fresh | ☺ | Free of lactose. |
| Peach, fresh | ☺ | Free of lactose. |

| Fruit | LACTOSE | Standard amount | |
|---|---|---|---|
| Pear, fresh | ☺ | Free of lactose. | |
| Persimmon, fresh | ☺ | Free of lactose. | |
| Pineapple, dried | ☺ | Free of lactose. | |
| Pineapple, fresh | ☺ | Free of lactose. | |
| Plantains, green, boiled | ☺ | Free of lactose. | |
| Plum, fresh | ☺ | Free of lactose. | |
| Pomegranate, fresh (arils-seed/juice sacs) | ☺ | Free of lactose. | |
| Quince, fresh | ☺ | Free of lactose. | |
| Raisins, uncooked | ☺ | Free of lactose. | |
| Rambutan, canned in syrup | ☺ | Free of lactose. | |
| Raspberries, fresh, red | ☺ | Free of lactose. | |
| Rhubarb, fresh | ☺ | Free of lactose. | |
| Rose hips | ☺ | Free of lactose. | |
| Santa Claus melon | ☺ | Free of lactose. | |
| Sapodilla, fresh | ☺ | Free of lactose. | |
| Sour cherries, fresh | ☺ | Free of lactose. | |

| Fruit | LACTOSE | Standard amount | |
|-------|---------|-----------------|---|
| Soursop (guanabana), fresh | ☺ | Free of lactose. | |
| Strawberries, fresh | ☺ | Free of lactose. | |
| Sweet cherries, fresh | ☺ | Free of lactose. | |
| Watermelon, fresh | ☺ | Free of lactose. | |

# 3.7.2   Vegetables

| Vegetables | LACTOSE | Standard amount | |
|---|---|---|---|
| Alfalfa sprouts | 😃 | Free of lactose. | |
| Artichoke, globe raw | 😃 | Free of lactose. | |
| Arugula, raw | 😃 | Free of lactose. | |
| Asparagus, raw | 😃 | Free of lactose. | |
| Avocado, green skin, Florida type | 😃 | Free of lactose. | |
| Bamboo shoots, canned and drained | 😃 | Free of lactose. | |
| Beets, raw | 😃 | Free of lactose. | |
| Black beans, cooked from dried | 😃 | Free of lactose. | |
| Black olives | 😃 | Free of lactose. | |
| Bok choy, raw | 😃 | Free of lactose. | |
| Boston Market® sweet corn | 😃 | Free of lactose. | |
| Broccoflower (green cauliflower), cooked from fresh | 😃 | Free of lactose. | |
| Broccoli, raw | 😃 | Free of lactose. | |
| Brown mushrooms (Italian or Crimini mushrooms), raw | 😃 | Free of lactose. | |
| Brussels sprouts, cooked from fresh | 😃 | Free of lactose. | |

| Vegetables | LACTOSE | Standard amount |
|---|---|---|
| Cabbage, green, cooked | 🙂 | Free of lactose. |
| Cabbage, red, cooked | 🙂 | Free of lactose. |
| Cabbage, savoy, raw | 🙂 | Free of lactose. |
| Carrots, cooked from fresh | 🙂 | Free of lactose. |
| Carrots, raw | 🙂 | Free of lactose. |
| Cauliflower, cooked from frozen | 🙂 | Free of lactose. |
| Celeriac (celery root), cooked from fresh | 🙂 | Free of lactose. |
| Celery, cooked | 🙂 | Free of lactose. |
| Chard, raw or blanched, marinated in oil | 🙂 | Free of lactose. |
| Chayote squash, cooked | 🙂 | Free of lactose. |
| Chestnuts, boiled, steamed | 🙂 | Free of lactose. |
| Chicory coffee powder, unprepared | 🙂 | Free of lactose. |
| Chicory greens, raw | 🙂 | Free of lactose. |
| Coleslaw, with apples and raisins, mayo dressing | 🙂 | Free of lactose. |
| Coleslaw, with pineapple, mayo dressing | 🙂 | Free of lactose. |
| Collards, raw | 🙂 | Free of lactose. |

| Vegetables | LACTOSE | Standard amount |
|---|---|---|
| Cucumber, raw, with peel | ☺ | Free of lactose. |
| Cucumber, raw, without peel | ☺ | Free of lactose. |
| Eggplant, cooked | ☺ | Free of lactose. |
| Endive, curly, raw | ☺ | Free of lactose. |
| Enoki mushrooms, raw | ☺ | Free of lactose. |
| Fennel bulb, raw | ☺ | Free of lactose. |
| Garbanzo beans (chickpeas), canned, drained | ☺ | Free of lactose. |
| Garlic, fresh | ☺ | Free of lactose. |
| Ginger root, raw | ☺ | Free of lactose. |
| Green beans (string beans), cooked from fresh | ☺ | Free of lactose. |
| Green bell peppers | ☺ | Free of lactose. |
| Green olives | ☺ | Free of lactose. |
| Green tomato, raw | ☺ | Free of lactose. |
| Grits (polenta), regular cooking | ☺ | Free of lactose. |
| Hot chili peppers, green, cooked from fresh | ☺ | Free of lactose. |
| Hot chili peppers, red, cooked from fresh | ☺ | Free of lactose. |

| Vegetables | LACTOSE | Standard amount |
|---|---|---|
| Hubbard squash | ☺ | Free of lactose. |
| Jerusalem artichoke (sun-choke), raw | ☺ | Free of lactose. |
| Kale, raw | ☺ | Free of lactose. |
| Kelp, raw | ☺ | Free of lactose. |
| Kidney beans, cooked from dried | ☺ | Free of lactose. |
| Kohlrabi, cooked | ☺ | Free of lactose. |
| Leeks, leafs | ☺ | Free of lactose. |
| Leeks, root | ☺ | Free of lactose. |
| Leeks, whole | ☺ | Free of lactose. |
| Lentils, cooked from dried | ☺ | Free of lactose. |
| Lettuce, Boston, bibb or butter-head | ☺ | Free of lactose. |
| Lettuce, green leaf | ☺ | Free of lactose. |
| Lettuce, iceberg | ☺ | Free of lactose. |
| Lettuce, red leaf | ☺ | Free of lactose. |
| Lettuce, romaine or cos | ☺ | Free of lactose. |
| Lima beans, cooked from dried | ☺ | Free of lactose. |

| Vegetables | LACTOSE | Standard amount | |
|---|---|---|---|
| Lotus root, cooked | 😊 | Free of lactose. | |
| Maitake mushrooms, raw | 😊 | Free of lactose. | |
| Morel mushrooms, raw | 😊 | Free of lactose. | |
| Mung bean sprouts, cooked from fresh | 😊 | Free of lactose. | |
| Mung beans, cooked from dried | 😊 | Free of lactose. | |
| Mushrooms, batter dipped or breaded | 😊 | Free of lactose. | |
| Okra, raw | 😊 | Free of lactose. | |
| Onion, white, yellow or red, raw | 😊 | Free of lactose. | |
| Oyster mushrooms, raw | 😊 | Free of lactose. | |
| Parsnip, cooked | 😊 | Free of lactose. | |
| Pickled beets | 😊 | Free of lactose. | |
| Portabella mushrooms, cooked from fresh | 😊 | Free of lactose. | |
| Purslane, raw | 😊 | Free of lactose. | |
| Radicchio, raw | 😊 | Free of lactose. | |
| Radish, raw | 😊 | Free of lactose. | |
| Rutabaga, raw or blanched, marinated in oil mixture | 😊 | Free of lactose. | |

| Vegetables | LACTOSE | Standard amount |
|---|---|---|
| Sauerkraut | 😊 | Free of lactose. |
| Scallop squash | 😊 | Free of lactose. |
| Shallot, raw | 😊 | Free of lactose. |
| Shiitake mushrooms, cooked | 😊 | Free of lactose. |
| Snow peas (edible pea pods), cooked from fresh | 😊 | Free of lactose. |
| Sour pickles | 😊 | Free of lactose. |
| Soybean sprouts, raw | 😊 | Free of lactose. |
| Soybeans, cooked from dried | 😊 | Free of lactose. |
| Spaghetti squash | 😊 | Free of lactose. |
| Spinach, cooked from fresh | 😊 | Free of lactose. |
| Split pea sprouts, cooked | 😊 | Free of lactose. |
| Straw mushrooms, canned, drained | 😊 | Free of lactose. |
| Summer squash, cooked from fresh | 😊 | Free of lactose. |
| Sun-dried tomatoes, oil pack, drained | 😊 | Free of lactose. |
| Sweet potato, boiled | 😊 | Free of lactose. |
| Tempeh | 😊 | Free of lactose. |

| Vegetables | LACTOSE | Standard amount |
|---|---|---|
| Tomato, cooked from fresh | 🙂 | Free of lactose. |
| Turnip, cooked | 🙂 | Free of lactose. |
| Wax beans (yellow beans), canned, drained | 🙂 | Free of lactose. |
| Winter melon (waxgourd or chinese preserving melon) | 🙂 | Free of lactose. |
| Winter type (dark green or orange) squash, cooked | 🙂 | Free of lactose. |
| Yams, sweet potato type, boiled | 🙂 | Free of lactose. |
| Yellow bell pepper, raw | 🙂 | Free of lactose. |
| Yellow tomato, raw | 🙂 | Free of lactose. |

# 3.8 Ice cream

| Ice cream | LACTOSE | | Standard amount | |
|---|---|---|---|---|
| Ben & Jerry's® Ice Cream, Brownie Batter | ¼ | | Portion (110g); 28g in total. | +¼ |
| Ben & Jerry's® Ice Cream, Chocolate Chip Cookie Dough | ½ | | Portion (104g); 52g in total. | +¼ |
| Ben & Jerry's® Ice Cream, Chubby Hubby® | ½ | | Portion (107g); 54g in total. | +½ |
| Ben & Jerry's® Ice Cream, Chunky Monkey® | ¼ | | Portion (107g); 27g in total. | +¼ |
| Ben & Jerry's® Ice Cream, Half Baked | ¼ | | Portion (108g); 27g in total. | +¼ |
| Ben & Jerry's® Ice Cream, Karamel Sutra® | ½ | | Portion (106g); 53g in total. | +¼ |
| Ben & Jerry's® Ice Cream, New York Super Fudge Chunk® | ½ | | Portion (106g); 53g in total. | +½ |
| Ben & Jerry's® Ice Cream, One Sweet Whirled | ½ | | Portion (106g); 53g in total. | +¼ |
| Ben & Jerry's® Ice Cream, Peanut Butter Cup | ½ | | Portion (115g); 58g in total. | +¼ |
| Ben & Jerry's® Ice Cream, Phish Food® | ¼ | | Portion (104g); 26g in total. | +¼ |
| Ben & Jerry's® Ice Cream, Vanilla For A Change | ½ | | Portion (103g); 52g in total. | +¼ |
| Breyers® Ice Cream, Natural Vanilla, Lactose Free | 4 | | Portion (65g); 260g in total. | +3¼ |
| Dreyer's® Grand Ice Cream, Chocolate | 1 | | Portion (65g); 65g in total. | +1 |
| Dreyer's® No Sugar Added Ice Cream, Triple Chocolate | 11½ | | Tsp. (5g); 58g in total. | +9½ |

| Ice cream | LACTOSE | Standard amount | |
|---|---|---|---|
| Drumstick® (sundae cone) | 1 | Piece (96g); 96g in total. | +¾ |
| Frozen fruit juice Bar | ☺ | Free of lactose. | |
| Haagen-Dazs® Desserts Extraordinaire Ice Cream, Creme Brulee | ½ | Portion (107g); 54g in total. | +¼ |
| Haagen-Dazs® Frozen Yogurt, chocolate or coffee flavors | ½ | Portion (106g); 53g in total. | +½ |
| Haagen-Dazs® Frozen Yogurt, vanilla or other flavors | ½ | Portion (106g); 53g in total. | +½ |
| Haagen-Dazs® Ice Cream, Bailey's Irish Cream | ½ | Portion (102g); 51g in total. | +¼ |
| Haagen-Dazs® Ice Cream, Black Walnut | ½ | Portion (106g); 53g in total. | +½ |
| Haagen-Dazs® Ice Cream, Butter Pecan | ½ | Portion (106g); 53g in total. | +½ |
| Haagen-Dazs® Ice Cream, Cherry Vanilla | ½ | Portion (101g); 51g in total. | +½ |
| Haagen-Dazs® Ice Cream, Chocolate | ¼ | Portion (106g); 27g in total. | +¼ |
| Haagen-Dazs® Ice Cream, Coffee | ¼ | Portion (106g); 27g in total. | +¼ |
| Haagen-Dazs® Ice Cream, Cookies & Cream | ½ | Portion (102g); 51g in total. | +¼ |
| Haagen-Dazs® Ice Cream, Mango | ¼ | Portion (106g); 27g in total. | +¼ |
| Haagen-Dazs® Ice Cream, Pistachio | ½ | Portion (106g); 53g in total. | +½ |
| Haagen-Dazs® Ice Cream, Rocky Road | ¼ | Portion (104g); 26g in total. | +¼ |

| Ice cream | LACTOSE | | Standard amount | |
|---|---|---|---|---|
| Haagen-Dazs® Ice Cream, Strawberry | ½ | | Portion (106g); 53g in total. | +¼ |
| Haagen-Dazs® Ice Cream, Vanilla Chocolate Chip | ½ | | Portion (106g); 53g in total. | +½ |
| Ice cream sandwich | 1¼ | | Piece (72g); 90g in total. | +1 |
| Ice cream, light, no sugar added, with aspartame, vanilla or other flavors (include chocolate chip) | 9¾ | | Tsp. (5g); 49g in total. | +8 |
| Popsicle | | | Free of lactose. | |
| Popsicle, sugar free | | | Free of lactose. | |
| Sorbet, chocolate | | | Nearly free of lactose | |
| Sorbet, coconut | 18¾ | | Portion (106g); 1988g in total. | +15½ |
| Sorbet, fruit | | | Free of lactose. | |

## 3.9   Ingredients

| Ingredients | LACTOSE | | Standard amount | ⊖ |
|---|---|---|---|---|
| Baking powder | | 😊 | Free of lactose. | |
| Barley flour | | 😊 | Free of lactose. | |
| Lemon peel | | 😊 | Free of lactose. | |
| Orange peel | | 😊 | Free of lactose. | |
| Rye flour,in recipes not containing yeast | | 😊 | Free of lactose. | |
| Semolina flour | | 😊 | Free of lactose. | |
| Spelt flour | | 😊 | Free of lactose. | |
| Streusel topping, crumb | 68¼ | 🍽 | Portion (19.56g); 1335g in total. | +57 |
| Wheat bran, unprocessed | | 😊 | Free of lactose. | |
| White all-purpose flour, unenriched | | 😊 | Free of lactose. | |
| White whole wheat flour | | 😊 | Free of lactose. | |

# Glossary

| Abbreviation | Meaning |
|---|---|
| EFSA | European Food Safety Authority. |
| FDA | Food and Drug Administration. |
| Fructans | Quickly fermentable carbohydrates that are contained in grain products for example. Included in this group are inulin, kestose and nystose. |
| Fructose | Oligosaccharide that is primarily contained in fruit. |
| Galactans | Quickly fermentable carbohydrates that are contained in beans, cabbage, lentils and peas for example (raffinose and stachyose). |
| Hereditary fructose intolerance | This disease is rare. If you are affected, fructose has a poisonous effect on you. Only a specialist can find out if you are affected and you have to check it before doing a test for fructose intolerance, as it could otherwise be lethal. |
| Irritable bowel | Definition of this book: an irritable bowel is one that reacts much more intensely to indigestions than it is commonly the case. The presence of trigger cubes in the intestine triggers the symptoms. |
| Lactose | Oligosaccharide that is primarily contained in dairy products. |
| Meal | One of three main meals of a given day. The first meal happens at about 7 am the second one at about 1 pm and the third one at about 7 pm. Hence, between each meal there has to be a gap of about six hours in order to avoid overloading your enzyme workers. The tolerable portion sizes refer to this definition of a meal. |
| NCC | Nutrition Coordination Center of the University of Minnesota. |

| Abbreviation | Meaning |
|---|---|
| Sensitivity level | Aside from the standard level, you can use multipliers to determine portion sizes in case you are less sensitive. In the LAXIBA app, we have calculated the tolerable amounts for you. Before increasing your portion sizes to fit another level, you should do a level test to check, if you can tolerate the higher load. There are four levels, see Chapter 3.1.3. |
| Sorbitol | Sugar alcohol. Although we should talk about a sugar alcohol sensitivity one usually refers to it as a sorbitol intolerance, because sorbitol is best known. |
| Standard | Portion sizes in this column are based on the usual sensitivity in case of an intolerance towards tlactose, i.e. as long as you consume less than the stated maximum amount for this level, you are likely to be untroubled by symptoms from it. It only applies in case of intolerance or certain test phases. Note that if you consume the maximum portion size for a food at a meal, you cannot eat any other foods that contain the cube at that meal. To combine two foods that contain a certain cube you have to reduce the stated portion sizes accordingly, e.g. by dividing both by two. |
| Sugar alcohols | These are contained in some fruit, like apples. Moreover, they are part of many diabetic, dietary and light products as well as chewing gums and mints. They are not contained in stevia. Part of the group of sugar alcohols besides sorbitol are erythritol, inositol, isomalt, lactitol, maltitol, mannitol, pinitol and xylitol. |
| Trigger(cube)s | Carbohydrates that fermented in the intestine. To this group belong oligosaccharides (fructose, fructans and galactans, lactose) and sugar-alcohols (like sorbitol). |

# 4

# ADVANCED PROCEDURES

## 4.1 Level test

| | Level test tasks | ✔ |
|---|---|---|
| **1** | You filled out the symptom test sheet for the status quo check. | ✔ |
| **2** | You asked your doctor to refer you to a specialist to do a breath test (if available). | ✔ |
| **3** | You performed the three-week introductory diet and found an improvement to your symptoms at the efficiency check (otherwise get *THE IBS NAVIGATOR* and find your trigger). If no breath test was available, you performed the substitute test. | ✔ |
| **4** | Now you convince a partner to help you with your tests. Alternatively, you book a personal trainer at *https://laxiba.com/trainer*. The partner will mix your test liquids and interpret your symptom test sheets. You can count on their confidentiality, credibility and availability. | |
| **5** | You finished all of the tests, during which your testing partner adhered to the instructions on page 181, and you acted according to the flowchart on page 192. | |
| **6** | Finish: You talked your result over with your testing partner, and adapted your serving sizes to your sensitivity level. | |

Each human differs in the amount he or she can stomach of each trigger. Even in healthy humans the tolerated amount of lactose fluctuates. Moreover, the amount consumed at once for the breath or substitute test is higher than what you would consume in a typical meal. Hence, if your enzyme-workers were able to cope with that amount—you were spared from symptoms after consuming the test does—you can be proud of them, and you can give them a positive interim report: They have mastered all tasks for lactose with flying colors.

If your crew has ached at the dose, at that point all we know is that the extreme test amount has been too much for them. What it does not mean is that the standard portion sizes used in this book are the highest load your enzyme workers can take. Where is your personal threshold up to which you will not have symptoms? To determine it, you use the level test described in the following. With it, you challenge your enzyme worker gradually and check your sensitivity. With each step, you increase the consumption amount of lactose up to the point at which your enzyme workers ask for a pay raise. The flowchart on page 192 on depicts the procedure.

For the level test, you ideally have a test partner preparing the test liquids for you and checking the results. If you have one, only let your partner read the instructions on the pages 177 onward. To increase the reliability, you test each level twice. Otherwise, chance could cause something else to trigger your symptom. Should you consider the matter too private and rather not have someone else included, follow the instructions for self-testers you find on those pages.

Start your test week three days before the test day, as symptoms may occur as many as three days after you consume lactose containing foods, and you want to start the check uninfluenced from "old" symptoms. On the days before the test, eat according to your current level. Your current level is the one that you tolerated during the test and retest of the last test. Initially, it is the level 1 on which the standard serving sizes in the food tables of Chapter 3 are based on.

## How to run a test week

| Day 1–3 before the test day | On the test day | Day 1–3 after |
|---|---|---|
| Your cube consumption should undercut your current lactose levels by as narrow a margin as possible, but do not force yourself to eat more of anything than you want. If you do not feel as well on the morning of the test day as you did at the end of the introductory diet, reschedule the test until you do. | Fill out the symptom test sheet on the test day and its three subsequent days. | |
| | At breakfast, lunch and dinner consume the level dose and apart from that avoid lactose-containing foods. | Eat accoding to the level on day 1-3 before the test. Hence, if you test level 2go back down to level 1. |

**Acceleration option:** Perform the tests right after one another. Three days after the last test day, begin the next test day and thus save the three days described in the column on the left.

You do not have to fill out the symptom test sheet during the days leading up to the test (page 27). Instead, you can use the efficiency check sheet as your reference, but from the day of the test to the third day after it, document your symptoms (unless you determine an intolerance earlier).

When your testing partner confirms you have an intolerance, the level test is over. You can find the precise procedure in the flowcharts in Section 4.2. For procedural reasons, wait until after you have repeated the test before trying to interpret the results.

## How to handle symptoms

**After** noting discomforts that were so severe that you told your test collaborate you malabsorbed the load, drink water (up to three liters per day are usually healthy) and take a walk to reduce your symptoms.

## Information for your level test partner:

| | | |
|---|---|---|
| Beginn the tolerance test with | ☐ Level 1 | ☐ Level 2 |
| My calculated K.O. threshold grade is: | | |

Some keep half the standard amounts at the introductory diet and then test level 1, because they consider themselves more sensible than other with lactose intolerance—mark that in case. If you want to use the mathematical Option B, presented at the end of this Chapter or are using our downloadable tool, enter your K.O.-grade from the efficiency check above or give your partner the filled out excel sheets. Important: disregard triggers that you can stomach—you can consume products containing them just as you did before. Background: if your estimated symptom grade (lid value) after a level test is lower or equal to the estimate K.O. grade, you have tolerated the test load and thereby the level and otherwise you have not.

 ## Summary

**As part of the strategy, you first performed the introductory diet to find out, if the diet did reduce your symptoms after all. If it had an effect, you can go on to determine your individual sensitivity to avoid unnecessary restrictions.**

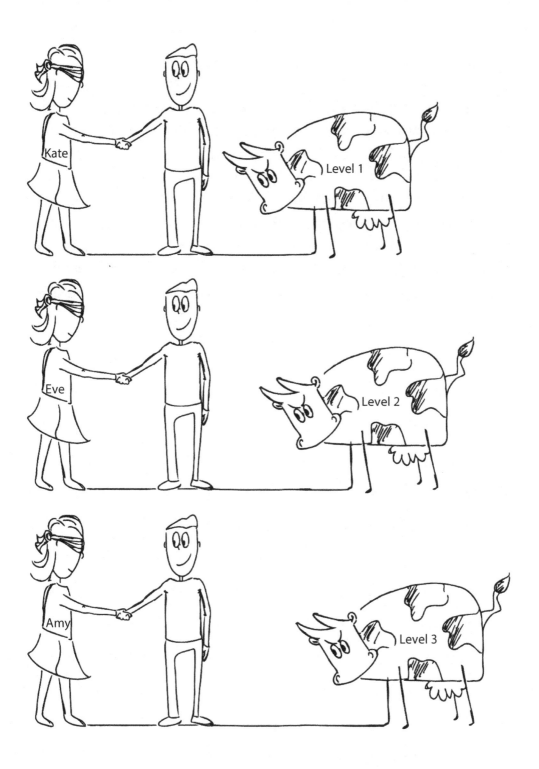

**Everyone's sensitivity level is different.**

**STOP:** The following pages are for only your testing partner to read, as they contain information regarding procedural safety—unless you want to do the test alone! Your partner's instructions will depend on your reactions; if you know how your partner is assessing you, you may alter your behavior and distort the results. Continue reading on page 192 to learn about the procedure underlying your partner's tolerance statements. Before and after the three pages for your testing partner are four empty pages. Thus, you can flick back from the end of the book to arrive at page 192 without reading them.

The **instructions** for your testing **partner** follow on page **181**. As the **reader** of the book, you should leave them **unread**, to **produce** a **more accurate** test **result**. Hence, open a new page that is farther **ahead** and then **flick back** to page **192**.

The **instructions** for your testing **partner** follow on page **181**. As the **reader** of the book, you should leave them **unread**, to **produce** a **more accurate** test **result**. Hence, open a new page that is much farther **ahead** and then **flick back** to page **192**.

The **instructions** for your testing **partner** follow on page **181**. As the **reader** of the book, you should leave them **unread**, to **produce** a **more accurate** test **result**. Hence, open a new page that is much farther **ahead** and then **flick back** to page **192**.

The **instructions** for your testing **partner** follow on page **181**. As the **reader** of the book, you should leave them **unread**, to **produce** a **more accurate** test **result**. Hence, open a new page that is much farther **ahead** and then **flick back** to page **192**.

**Your friend needs your help! Instructions for testing partners:**

You are not the testing partner but the aggrieved party? In case, I caught you! However, of course you also find instructions how to conduct the test yourself. If have a testing partner these lines are not for you, would you please finally move on to page 192!

Now we are in private. Your friend cannot stomach the common food ingredient lactose and wants to find out about the personal tolerance limit. Unfortunately, a placebo effect is quite common in this test. Your role in this test is critical for avoiding a false result. You are going to do two rounds per level, each test taking about a week. On one of the two days, you are going to hand out a placebo mix instead of the real one. Your friend does not know about the placebo. Just say that the double test is required to get valid results, as you also have to keep track of certain behaviors she or he might exhibit. IMPORTANT: Keep quiet about the placebo until **all** tests are done (use the flowchart on page 192) and you have talked the results over. Waiting until the end of that final discussion is important, as your friend may want to test another level as well. Between two test days are three monitoring days and three regeneration days. Here is what you need: a beaker, a letter scale, and three 0.5 L bottles. Also, instruct your friend to stop taking another bottle if the symptoms after drinking one are already indicating that the load was too much.

> **Note for a test without testing partner**: Prepare the required test bottles on the eve before the test. Make the real and the placebo mix in an equal looking 1-liter-bottle with a non-transparent plastic label (the foil around the bottle on which the brand name shows up). If you use milk, make sure it is still usable for at least two weeks. Now use a pen and write placebo on a colored memo, fold it twice to form a smaller square and put it behind the label of the bottle with the placebo mix. On another note in the same color, you write real mix and put it behind the label of the other bottle. Then you put sticky tape around the tags. Then put both bottles into a non-transparent box that is longer, wider and higher than the bottles. Close it and then turn it around ten times. Thus, you have successfully outwitted yourself: put the bottles in the fridge! On the next morning, you take out one of the bottles, mark it with 1 and drink one third of the mixture in the morning, one third at lunchtime and the rest of the evening (you use one bottle with the daily amount instead of three here, according to the first column of the following tables).

If you find yourself trying to spy at the memo, give yourself a slap on the finger. After the three days following it, where you observed your symptoms, you repeat the test with the other bottle. Again, no fiddling with the label! You have to wait with that until the three observance days of the second bottle are over, too. Now check, how you stomached the placebo versus the real mix.

If your friend has not given you the substances for the test solution, you can order them online or from a pharmacy. You can also ask your pharmacist to weigh the amounts you need. From test to test, increase the level amounts according to the table on the following page. Begin with the level 2. Before repeating the test, note whether you first handed out the real or placebo mix and the result. Ideally, you should ask for the symptom test sheet and write down L for reaL and A for plAcebo as well as the result. Then, keep all of the info sheets for the final discussion of all tests. If your friend has given you the K-grade, you can calculate the tolerance (see row L on page 194). If the L-grade is greater than or equal to K, this indicates an intolerance. There are three possible cases after each double test:

**Case 1:** Neither the placebo nor the real mix causes the symptoms to worsen, i.e., your friend can stomach the amounts of the ingredient, and you can test the next level. Tell her/him that.

**Case 2:** Only the real mix causes the symptoms to worsen, i.e., your friend is intolerant for the amount. The test series is over, and you can tell your friend.

**Case 3:** The placebo mix causes symptoms to worsen. Regardless of whether or not the real mix causes symptoms to worsen, as well, repeat the test with the same amount, starting with the placebo mix, but tell her that you reduced the amount to half of the dose. If your friend still reports an intolerance, abort the test and tell her/him that s/he has an intolerance for the amount, and the old levels remain current.

After the test and retest of the first level, continue according to the level test flowchart on pp. 192. On the eve of one of the two test days, hand out three bottles with the real mix, and on the other one, three bottles with the placebo. At breakfast, lunch and dinner your friend drinks one bottle. Find the mixtures for each level in the following explanation and table.

In the **left column** find the respective **level** and the **total amount** of substances per day, as it is easier to mix the **daily amount in one load** and **then divide** it among the **three bottles**. In the two columns on the right, find the amounts per bottle for the real/placebo substance. Required: 1 L reduced-fat milk, 1 L lactose-free cow milk, and vanilla extract. To hide taste differences between the regular, and the lactose-free milk, please add a little bit of vanilla extract (**v.**) to both.

| **Level** and lactose amount as well as milk **sum/day** | Real (R) 3 × bottle with | Placebo (P) 3 × bottle with |
|---|---|---|
| **Level 1** (3g/meal) per day 180 mL milk and ½ tsp. of **v.** | 4 tbsp. (60 mL) milk 1 drop of **v.** | 4 tbsp. lactose-free milk 1 drop of **v.** |
| **Level 2** (6g/meal) per day 360 mL milk and ¾ tsp. of **v.** | 120 mL milk (100) 2 drops of **v.** | 120 mL lactose-free milk 2 drops of **v.** |
| **Level 3** (9g/meal) per day 540 mL milk and 1 tsp. of **v.** | 180 mL milk 3 drops of **v.** | 180 mL lactose-free milk 3 drops of **v.** |

Thank you very much for your support! Even if you have to overcome scruples to knowingly trick your friend… You do not? Well then, enjoy the white lie for good reason!

The **instructions** for your testing **partner** begin on page **181**. As the **reader** of the book, you should leave them **unread**, to **produce** a **more accurate** test **result**. The book resumes on page 192.

The **instructions** for your testing **partner** begin on page **181**. As the **reader** of the book, you should leave them **unread**, to **produce** a **more accurate** test **result**. The book resumes on page 192.

The **instructions** for your testing **partner** begin on page **181**. As the **reader** of the book, you should leave them **unread**, to **produce** a **more accurate** test **result**. The book resumes on page 192.

The **instructions** for your testing **partner** begin on page **181**. As the **reader** of the book, you should leave them **unread**, to **produce** a **more accurate** test **result**.

# 4.2　Symptom-based test process

The following flow charts shows you the next step, depending on your reaction to the test load. Remember, if you have symptoms after taking the first of three test loads on a test day, abort the test—as this shows that the tested sensitivity level is too high, and there is no point in tantalizing yourself.

You start the test with the first field of the flow chart. The next step always depends on your test result. If you did not stomach a load, the test is over, and you should stick to the level below, which you did tolerate—at the beginning this is the standard amount in the tables in Chapter 3.

All statements assume that you want to perform the level test to the highest level. However, maybe, it is enough to you to know if you tolerate the next level, in the case just stop after the first test. If you do tolerate more than the standard level, note your level next to the multipliers, see Chapter 3.1.3. You will also be able to select your level when using our mobile phone application. Attention: During the combined level tests, you must not pass any level amount that holds for one of your triggers that you do not check at the time as this may otherwise distort the result. If it does happen, you have to repeat the check.

# Lactose-level-test

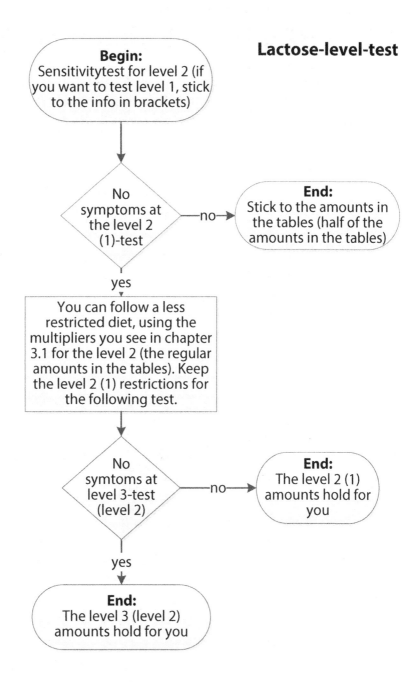

**Begin:**
Sensitivitytest for level 2 (if you want to test level 1, stick to the info in brackets)

**No symptoms at the level 2 (1)-test**

—no→ **End:**
Stick to the amounts in the tables (half of the amounts in the tables)

yes

You can follow a less restricted diet, using the multipliers you see in chapter 3.1 for the level 2 (the regular amounts in the tables). Keep the level 2 (1) restrictions for the following test.

**No symtoms at level 3-test (level 2)**

—no→ **End:**
The level 2 (1) amounts hold for you

yes

**End:**
The level 3 (level 2) amounts hold for you

# 4.3   Test result calculation table

You have two calculation options: option **A** is slightly simpler than option **B**. Real cracks immediately start with **B**. **B** saves time at any further check, and you get a statement on your tolerance. [2]

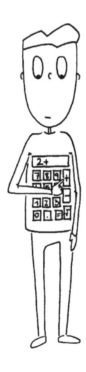

---

[2] From a statistical point of view the survey is slim and the result vague.

# 4.3.1   The efficiency check calculation table

You use the following table and enter the total intensity of bloating of the respective day into the row **A**. Into the first four cells of that row, you enter the results of the **efficiency check days**, i.e. the last days of your introductory diet. Into the remaining four fields of that row, you enter the values of the **status-quo-days** (the four days before starting your introductory diet, hence, before reducing your trigger consumption).

**Calculation option A**: Determine $A1$ = total stool grade at the first day of your efficiency check, i.e. your grade in the morning (you calculate your stool grade by multiplying your stool value by the number of defecations you had in the morning) plus the grade at lunchtime plus the grade at the evening. Likewise, you proceed with all other **A**-numbers. Afterward, you determine the **B**-numbers: $B1 = A1$ plus the bloating grade at the first efficiency-check-day plus the pain grade on that day. You calculate $B2$ likewise with the grades for day 2 and so on. Next, you calculate $C2$ and afterward $D2$, which is the average of the status-quo-check-days. To interpret the result, you compare $D2$ with the highest day-grade of the efficiency-check-days, the highest grade of the group $B1$ to $B4$. When checking the success of the introductory diet, it holds that the greater $D2$ lies above the maximum grade of the group the more likely it is that the introductory diet was successful in lowering your symptoms.

**Calculation Option B:** You calculate $A1$ to $A8$ as well as $B1$ to $B8$ according to the calculation option **A**. Afterward, you estimate $C1$ and $D1$, as well as $C2$ and $D2$ and proceed with the steps described in the table up to $K$. To interpret the result you compare the $D2$-value with the $K$-value, i.e. the K. O.[3] threshold grade. At the introductory diet, it holds that: If $D2$ is bigger or equal to the $K$-grade; this indicates that the diet successfully lowered your symptoms.

If the diet fails, however, try sensitivity level zero and otherwise get *THE IBS NAVIGATOR* and perform a substitute test for fructans and galactans or check alternative triggers as described there.

.

---

[3] K = if L tops this K.-O.-threshold, the level test amount is too much for your enzyme workers.

| | Efficiency check day- | | | | Status-quo-check-day before introductory diet | | | |
|---|---|---|---|---|---|---|---|---|
| | **1:** | **2:** | **3:** | **4:** | **1:** | **2:** | **3:** | **4:** |
| **A** | A1 | A3 | A3 | A4 | A5 | A6 | A7 | A8 |

*Enter the total stool grade for each day into the A-cells*

| | | | | | | | | |
|---|---|---|---|---|---|---|---|---|
| **B** | B1 | B2 | B3 | B4 | B5 | B6 | B7 | B8 |

*B5 = stool- + bloating- + pain grade on status-quo-check-day 1*

| | | | |
|---|---|---|---|
| **C** | C1 | C1 = B1 + B2 + B3 + B4   Sum of cells B1 to B4 | C2 |
| | | C2 = B5 + B6 + B7 + B8   Sum of cells B5 to B8 | |
| **D** | D1 | D1 = C1 ÷ 4   Divide your result in cell C1 by 4 | D2 |
| | | D2 = C2 ÷ 4   Divide your result in cell C2 by 4 | |
| **E** | E1 | E2   E3   E4 | $E1 = B1 - D1$, $E2 = B2 - D1$ etc. To calculate E1, subtract D1 from B1. Negative results are possible. |
| **F** | F1 | F2   F3   F4 | $F1 = E1 \times E1$, $F2 = E2 \times E2$ etc. To calculate F1, multiply E1 by itself. As minus times minus is plus, all results are positive. |
| **G** | G | $G = F1 + F2 + F3 + F4$ Add your results of the cells F1 to F4 | |
| **H** | H | $H = G ÷ 4$ Divide G by 4 | |
| **I** | I | I = Take the root of H   Take the root of your result in H. On your calculator the root symbol looks like this: $\sqrt{\ }$. | |
| **J** | J | $J = I \times 2$ Multiply I by 2 | |
| **K** | K | $K = J + D1$ Add the result of cell J to the one in cell D1. The K-grade is the K. O. threshold grade as the success of the introductory diet depends on it. The diet lowered your symptoms if D2 is bigger than K ($D2 > K$). In addition, you can assess the success of the sensitivity level test with it. You tolerated the tested level if L is not bigger than K ($L \le K$). Please transfer the K-grade to the level test table. | |

# 1. Efficiency check calculation with page 29-30 values

| | Efficiency-check-day- | | | | Status-quo-check-day before introductory diet | | | |
|---|---|---|---|---|---|---|---|---|
| | 1: | 2: | 3: | 4: | 1: | 2: | 3: | 4: |
| **A** | A1 | A3 | A3 | A4 | A5 | | A6 | A7 | A8 |
| | 3 | 2 | 3 | 2 | | 16 | 14 | 12 | 14 |

*Enter the total stool grade for each day into the A-cells*

| | 1: | 2: | 3: | 4: | 1: | 2: | 3: | 4: |
|---|---|---|---|---|---|---|---|---|
| **B** | B1 | B2 | B3 | B4 | B5 | | B6 | B7 | B8 |
| | 9 | 8 | 11 | 8 | | 30 | 30 | 31 | 28 |

*B5 = stool- + bloating- + pain grade on status-quo-check-day 1*

| | | | |
|---|---|---|---|
| **C** | C1 | C1 = B1 + B2 + B3 + B4   Sum of cells B1 to B4 | C2 |
| | 36 | C2 = B5 + B6 + B7 + B8   Sum of cells B5 to B8 | 119 |
| **D** | D1 | D1 = C1 ÷ 4  Divide your result in cell C1 by 4 | D2 |
| | 9 | D2 = C2 ÷ 4  Divide your result in cell C2 by 4 | 29.75 |

| | 1: | 2: | 3: | 4: | |
|---|---|---|---|---|---|
| **E** | E1 | E2 | E3 | E4 | E1 = B1 - D1, E2 = B2 - D1 etc. |
| | | | | | To calculate E1, subtract D1 from B1. Negative |
| | 0 | -1 | 2 | -1 | results are possible. |
| **F** | F1 | F2 | F3 | F4 | F1 = E1 x E1, F2 = E2 x E2 etc. |
| | | | | | To calculate F1, multiply E1 by itself. As minus |
| | 0 | 1 | 4 | 1 | times minus is plus, all results are positive. |

| | | |
|---|---|---|
| **G** | G | G = F1 + F2 + F3 + F4 |
| | 6 | Add your results of the cells F1 to F4 |
| **H** | H | H = G ÷ 4 |
| | 1.5 | Divide G by 4 |
| **I** | I | I = Take the root of H   Take the root of your result in H. On your |
| | 1.22 | calculator the root symbol looks like this: √ . |
| **J** | J | J = I x 2 |
| | 2.45 | Multiply I by 2 |
| **K** | K | K = J + D1 |
| | | Add the result of cell J to the one in cell D1. The *K*-grade is called |
| | 11.45 | K. O. threshold grade as the success of the introductory diet (D2 > |
| | | K) and the sensitivity level test (L ≤ K) depend on it. |

## Calculation method A

D2 is 29.75 and thus way larger than the highest day grade, 11, (B3) of the group B1 to B4, which indicates the success of the introductory diet.

## Calculation method B

D2 = 29.75 is bigger than K = 11.45, and that shows the success of the diet. Had D2 been smaller or equal to K, try the diet at sensitivity level 0 (half the amount in the tables, or get *THE IBS NAVIGATOR* and check other potential triggers.

# 4.3.2 The level test calculation table

Use the following table and enter the grades of the level test days. You only need to estimate the grades from the level test sheet (enter them into B5 to B8. If you used math option B, just enter the K value, and you are ready to determine your result. If you use math option A, you have to calculate D1. Having done the introductory diet is, of course, necessary.

**Calculation option A**: *A1* = stool grade at the first efficiency-check-day, i.e. grade in the morning (multiply the stool value in the morning by the number of defecations you had in the morning) plus stool grade at lunchtime plus stool grade at the evening. Enter your total stool grade into the cell with the *A1* in italic. Likewise, you proceed with all other **A**-Numbers. Afterward, estimate the **B-grades**: *B1* = *A1* plus total bloating grade, plus total pain grade on the test day. You calculate *B2* with the grades for the first day after the test day and so on. Next, you determine *C1* and afterward *D1*, i.e. the average of the efficiency-check days. To interpret the result, compare *D1* with the highest day grade of the level test days, *B5* to *B8*. When checking the success of the diet, it holds that the much greater the largest day grade is compared to *D1*, the rather you did not tolerate the load of the tested sensitivity level. If that is the case, stick to the portion sizes of a lower sensitivity level.

**Calculation option B:** If you calculated *K* at the efficiency check—you should have as doing a level test before checking the efficiency of the diet makes no sense—just copy it to this table. Aside from it, all you need is to estimate *B1* to *B8* according to calculation option **A** and determine *L*. For the assessment, you compare the *L*-, i.e. the level grade with the *K*-grade, the K.-O.-threshold grade. It holds: if *L* is bigger than *K*, this means that the amount consumed during the test has triggered symptoms. Therefore, you should stick to the portion sizes of the sensitivity level below at which your symptoms improved. If *L* is lower than *K*, you tolerated the level amount and can have the less restricted diet according to that level. What is more, you can check an even higher sensitivity level if you want.

| Efficiency-check-day- | | | | Level-test | day after test day- | | |
|---|---|---|---|---|---|---|---|
| **1:** | **2:** | **3:** | **4:** | **Test day** | **1:** | **2:** | **3:** |
| **A** A1 | A3 | A3 | A4 | A5 | A6 | A7 | A8 |

*Enter the total stool grade for each day into the A-cells*

| | | | | | | | |
|---|---|---|---|---|---|---|---|
| **B** B1 | B2 | B3 | B4 | B5 | B6 | B7 | B8 |

*B5 = stool- + bloating- + pain grade on status-quo-check-day 1*

| | |
|---|---|
| **C** C1 | $C1 = B1 + B2 + B3 + B4$  Sum of the cells $B1$ to $B4$ |
| **D** D1 | $D1 = C1 \div 4$  Divide your results in cell $C1$ by 4 |
| **K** K | *Please copy the K grade you estimated at the end of the introductory diet to this field. If you have not yet calculated it, do it now as described in the efficiency-check-calculation-table.* |
| **L** L | $L$ = is the biggest grade of the group: $B5$, $B6$, $B7$, $B8$. This group contains the results of the level test day ($B5$) and the three days following it ($B6$ to $B8$). With the $L$-grade, you evaluate the current Level test. Assessment: $L > K$, if L is bigger than K, it means that the tested load for that level caused you symptoms and that you, therefore, should adjust your diet to a lower sensitivity level. $L \leq K$, if L is lower or equal to K, it means that you tolerated the load of that level per meal. |

# 1. Level test calculation with the page 29-30 values

| | Efficiency-check-day- | | | | Level-test | day after test day- | | |
|---|---|---|---|---|---|---|---|---|
| | **1:** | **2:** | **3:** | **4:** | **Test day** | **1:** | **2:** | **3:** |
| **A** | A1 | A3 | A3 | A4 | A5 | A6 | A7 | A8 |
| | 3 | 2 | 3 | 2 | 16 | 14 | 12 | 14 |

*Enter the total stool grade for each day into the A-cells*

| | **1:** | **2:** | **3:** | **4:** | **Test day** | **1:** | **2:** | **3:** |
|---|---|---|---|---|---|---|---|---|
| **B** | B1 | B2 | B3 | B4 | B5 | B6 | B7 | B8 |
| | 9 | 8 | 11 | 8 | 30 | 30 | 31 | 28 |

*B5 = stool- + bloating- + pain grade on status-quo-check-day 1*

| | | |
|---|---|---|
| **C** | C1 | $C1 = B1 + B2 + B3 + B4$  Sum of the cells B1 to B4 |
| | 36 | |
| **D** | D1 | $D1 = C1 \div 4$  Divide your results in cell C1 by 4 |
| | 9 | |
| **K** | K | *Please copy the K grade you estimated at the end of the introductory diet to this field. If you have not yet calculated it, do it now as described in the efficiency-check-calculation-table.* |
| | 11.45 | |
| **L** | L | $L$ = is the biggest grade of the group: B5, B6, B7, B8. This group contains the results of the level test day (B5) and the three days following it (B6 to B8). With the L-grade, you evaluate the current Level test. Assessment: |
| | | $L > K$, if L is bigger than K, it means that the tested load for that level caused you symptoms and that you, therefore, should adjust your diet to a lower sensitivity level. |
| | 31 | $L \leq K$, if L is lower or equal to K, it means that you tolerated the load of that level per meal. |

## Calculation method A

The highest total grade of a day of the group B5 to B8, B7 = 31 is way above D1 = 9, which indicates that you did not tolerate the level amount. If the highest grade of the group B5 to B8 had been smaller or equal to 9, you would have tolerated the sensitivity level amount and could have taken a less restricted diet according to the amounts of that level. Moreover, you could have tested the next level for people that are even less sensitive.

## Calculation method B

As L = 31 is bigger than K = 11.45, you have not tolerated the level load of that trigger. Had L been smaller or equal to 11.45, you would have endured the level amount and could have followed the less strict diet for that level. Moreover, you could have tested the next higher tolerance level.

# Sources

**Ali, M., Rellos, P., & Cox, T. M.** (1998). Heriditary fruktose intolerance. *Journal of Medical Genetics*, 35(5), 353-365.

**American Cancer Society** (2015). *Colorectal cancer and early detection*. Retrieved from: www.cancer.org/acs/groups/cis/documents/webcontent/003170-pdf.pdf.

**Ananthakrishnan, A. N., Higuchi, L. M., Huang, E. S., Khalili, H., Richter, J. M., Fuchs, C. S., & Chan, A. T.** (2012). Aspirin, nonsteroidal anti-inflammatory drug use, and risk for Crohn disease and ulcerative colitis: a cohort study. *Annals of Internal Medicine*, 156(5), 350-359.

**Barrett, J. S., Gearry, R. B., Muir, J. G., Irving, P. M., Rose, R., Rosella, O., ... & Gibson, P. R.** (2010). Dietary poorly absorbed, short-chain carbohydrates increase delivery of water and fermentable substrates to the proximal colon. *Alimentary Pharmacology & Therapeutics*, 31(8), 874-882.

**Balasubramanya, N. N., Sarwar, & Narayanan, K. M.** (1993). Effect of stage of lactation on oligosaccharides level in milk. *Indian Journal of Dairy & Biosciences*, 4, 58-60.

**Belitz, H.-D., Grosch, W., & Schieberle, P.** (2008). *Lehrbuch der Lebensmittelchemie* (6th ed.). Berlin Heidelberg: Springer.

**Berekoven, L., Eckert, W., Ellenrieder, P.** (2009). Marktforschung: *Methodische Grundlagen und praktische Anwendung* (12th ed.). Wiesbaden: Gabler.

**Bernstein, C. N., Fried, M., Krabshuis, J. H., Cohen, H., Eliakim, R., Fedail, S., ... & Watermeyer, G.** (2010). World Gastroenterology Organization Practice Guidelines for the diagnosis and management of IBD in 2010. *Inflammatory Bowel Diseases*, 16(1), 112-124.

**Biesiekierski, J. R., Rosella, O., Rose, R., Liels, K., Barrett, J. S., Shepherd, S. J., ... & Muir, J. G.** (2011). Quantification of fructans, galacto-oligosaccharides and other short-chain carbohydrates in processed grains and cereals. *Journal of Human Nutrition and Dietetics*, 24(2), 154-176.

**Binnendijk, K. H., & Rijkers, G. T.** (2013). What is a health benefit? An evaluation of EFSA opinions on health benefits with reference to probiotics. *Beneficial Microbes*, 4(3), 223-230.

**Blumenthal, M.** (1998). *The Complete German Commission E Monographs; Therapeutic Guide to Herbal Medicine*. Boston, MA: Integrative Medicine Communications.

**Boehm, G., & Stahl, B.** (2007). Oligosaccharides from milk. *The Journal of Nutrition*, 137(3), 847S-849S.

**Bowden, P.** (2011). *Telling It Like It Is*. Paul Bowden.

**Briançon, S., Boini, S., Bertrais, S., Guillemin, F., Galan, P., & Hercberg, S.** (2011). Long-term antioxidant supplementation has no effect on health-related quality of life: The randomized, double-blind, placebo-controlled, primary prevention SU.VI.MAX trial. *International Journal of Epidemiology*, 40(6), 1605-1616.

**Campbell, J. M., Fahey, G. C., & Wolf, B. W.** (1997). Selected indigestible oligosaccharides affect large bowel mass, cecal and fecal short-chain fatty acids, pH and microflora in rats. *The Journal of Nutrition*, 127(1), 130-136.

**Chi, W. J., Chang, Y. K., & Hong, S. K.** (2012). Agar degradation by microorganisms and agar-degrading enzymes. *Applied Microbiology and Biotechnology*, 94(4), 917-930.

**Choi, Y. K; Johlin Jr., F. C.; Summers, R.W., Jackson, M., & Rao, S. S. C.** (2003). Fruktose intolerance: an under-recognized problem. *The American Journal of Gastroenterology*, 98(6) 2003, S. 1348-1353.

**CIAA** (n. d.). *CIAA agreed reference values for GDAs* [Table]. Retrieved from http://gda.fooddrinkeurope.eu/asp2/gdas_portions_rationale.asp?doc_id=127.

**Connor, W. E.** (2000). Importance of n− 3 fatty acids in health and disease. *The American Journal of Clinical nutrition*, 71(1), 171S-175S.

**Coraggio, L.** (1990). *Deleterious Effects of Intermittent Interruptions on the Task Performance of Knowledge Workers: A Laboratory Investigation* (Doctoral Dissertation). Retrieved from http://arizona.openrepository.com.

**Corazza, G. R., Strocchi, A., Rossi, R., Sirola, D., & Fasbarrini, G.** (1988). Sorbitol malabsorption in normal volunteers and in patients with celiac disease. *Gut*, 29(1), 44-48.

**Cummings, J. H.** (1981). Short chain fatty acids in the human colon. *Gut*, 22(9), 763-779.

**Cummings, J. H., & Macfarlane, G. T.** (1997). Role of intestinal bacteria in nutrient metabolism. *Journal of Parental and Enteral Nutrition*, 21(6), 357-365.

**DGE** (2013). Vollwertig essen und trinken nach den 10 Regeln der DGE. 9th Edition, Bonn.

**Donker, G. A., Foets, M., & Spreeuwenberg, P.** (1999). Patients with irritable bowel syndrome: health status and use of healthcare services. *British Journal of General Practice*, 49(447), 787-792.

Drossman, D. A., Li, Z., Andruzzi, E., Temple, R. D., Talley, N. J., Thompson, W. G. ...Corazziari, E. et al. (1993). US householder survey of functional gastrointestinal disorders: prevalence, sociodemography, and health impact. *Digestive Diseases and Sciences*, 38(9), 1569-1580.

Dukas, L., Willett, W. C., & Giovannucci, E. L. (2003). Association between physical activity, fiber intake, and other lifestyle variables and constipation in a study of women. *The American Journal of Gastroenterology*, 98(8), 1790-1796.

EFSA (2007). Opinion of the scientific panel on dietetic products, nutrition and allergies on a request from the commission related to a notification from epa on lactitol pursuant to article 6, paragraph 11 of directive 2000/13/ec- for permanent exemption from labeling. *The EFSA Journal*, 5(10), 565-570.

EFSA (2012a). Scientific opinion on dietary reference values for protein. *The EFSA Journal*, 10(2), 2557-2622.

EFSA (2012b). Scientific opinion on the substantiation of health claims related to lactobacillus casei dg cncm i-1572 and decreasing potentially pathogenic gastro-intestinal microorganisms (id 2949, 3061, further assessment) pursuant to article 13(1) of regulation (ec) no 1924/2006. *The EFSA Journal*, 10(6), 2723-2637.

EFSA (2012c). Scientific opinion on the tolerable upper intake level of eicosapentaenoic acid (epa), docosahexaenoic acid (dha) and docosapentaenoic acid (dpa). *The EFSA Journal*, 10(7), 2815-2862.

EFSA (2013). scientific opinion on the substantiation of a health claim related to bimuno® gos and reducing gastro-intestinal discomfort pursuant to article 13(5) of regulation (ec) no 1924/2006. *The EFSA Journal*, 11(6), 3259-3268.

Eisenführ, F., Weber, M., & Langer, T. (2010): *Rational Decision Making*, Heidelberg, Berlin: Springer.

Erdman, K., Tunnicliffe, J., Lun, V. M., & Reimer, R. A. (2013). Eating patterns and composition of meals and snacks in elite canadian athletes. *International Journal Of Sport Nutrition & Exercise Metabolism*, 23(3), 210-219.

Evans, J. M., McMahon, A. D., Murray, F. E., McDevitt, D. G., & MacDonald, T. M. (1997). Non-steroidal anti-inflammatory drugs are associated with emergency admission to hospital for colitis due to inflammatory bowel disease. *Gut*, 40(5), 619-622.

Falony, G., Verschaeren, A. De Bruycker, F., De Preter, V., Verbecke, F. L., & De Vuyst L. (2009b). In vitro kinetics of prebiotic inulin-type fructan fermentation by butyrate-producing colon bacteria: implementation of online gas chromatography for quantitative analysis of carbon dioxide and hydrogen gas production. *Applied Environmental Microbiology*, 75(18), 5884-5892.

**FAO** (2008). Fats and fatty acids in human nutrition. *FAO Food and Nutrition Paper*, 91, 9-20.

**Farquhar, P. H., & Keller, L. R.** (1989). Preference intensity measurement. *Annals of Operations Research*, 19(1), 205-217.

**Farshchi, H. R., Taylor, M. A., & Macdonald, I. A.** (2004). Regular meal frequency creates more appropriate insulin sensitivity and lipid profiles compared with irregular meal frequency in healthy lean women. *European Journal of Clinical Nutrition*, 58(7), 1071-1077.

**Fasano, A., & Catassi, C.** (2001). Current approaches to diagnosis and treatment of celiac disease: an evolving spectrum. *Gastroenterology*, 120(3), 636-651.

**Fass, R., Fullerton, S., Naliboff, B., Hirsh, T., & Mayer, E. A.** (1998). Sexual dysfunction in patients with irritable bowel syndrom and non-ulcer dyspepsia. *Digestion*, 59(1), 79-85.

**Fernández-Bañares, F., Esteve-Pardo, M., de Leon, R., Humbert, P., Cabré, E., Llovet, J. M., & Gassull, M. A.** (1993). Sugar malabsorption in functional bowel disease: clinical implications. *American Journal of Gastroenterology*, 88(12), 2044-2050.

**Fox, K. (2013). N. t.. In Wells, V., Wyness, L., & Coe, S.** (Eds.). The British Nutrition Foundation's 45th anniversary conference: behaviour change in relation to healthier lifestyles. *Nutrition Bulletin*, 38(1), 100-107.

**Gaby, A. R.** (2005). Adverse effects of dietary fruktose. *Alternative medicine review*, 10(4).

**Gay-Crosier, F., Schreiber, G., & Hauser, C.** (2000). Anaphylaxis from inulin in vegetables and processed food. *The New England Journal of Medicine*, 342(18), 1372.

**German, J., Freeman, S., Lebrilla, C., & Mills, D.** (2008). Human milk oligosaccharides: evolution, structures and bioselectivity as substrates for intestinal bacteria, *Nestlé Nutrition Workshop, Pediatric Program*, 62, 205-222.

**Gibson, P. R., Newnham, E., Barrett, J. S., Shepherd, S. J., & Muir, J. G.** (2007). Review article: Fruktose malabsorption and the bigger picture. *Alimentary Pharmacology & Therapeutics*, 25(4), 349-363.

**Gibson, P. R., & Shepherd, S. J.** (2010). Evidence-based dietary management of functional gastrointestinal symptoms: the fodmap approach. *Journal of Gastroenterology and Hepatology*, 25(2), 252-258.

**Gilbert, P. (2013). N. t.. In Wells, V., Wyness, L., & Coe, S.** (Eds.). The British Nutrition Foundation's 45th anniversary conference: behaviour change in relation to healthier lifestyles. *Nutrition Bulletin*, 38(1), 100-107.

Goldstein, R., Braverman, D., & Stankiewicz, H. (2000). Carbohydrate malabsorption and the effect of dietary restriction on symptoms of irritable bowel syndrome and functional bowel complaints. *Israel Medical Association Journal*, 2(8), 583-587.

Gralnek, I. M., Hays, R. D., Kilbourne, A., Naliboff, B., & Mayer, E. A. (2000). The impact of irritable bowel syndrome on health-related quality of life. *Gastroenterology*, 119(3), 654-660.

Hahn, B. A., Kirchdoerfer, L. J., Fullerton, S., & Mayer, S. (1997). Patient perceived severity of irritable bowel syndrome in relation to symptoms, health resource utilization and quality of life. *Alimentary Pharmacology and Therapeutics*, 11(3), 553-559.

Hallert, C., Grant, C., Grehn, S., Grännö, C., Hultén, S., Midhagen, G., ... & Valdimarsson, T. (2002). Evidence of poor vitamin status in coeliac patients on a gluten-free diet for 10 years. *Alimentary Pharmacology & Therapeutics*, 16(7), 1333-1339.

Hanauer, S. B. (2006). Inflammatory bowel disease: epidemiology, pathogenesis, and therapeutic opportunities. *Inflammatory Bowel Diseases*, 12(5), S3-S9.

Hawthorne, B., Lambert, S., Scott, D., & Scott, B. (1991). Food intolerance and the irritable bowel syndrome. *Journal of Human Nutrition and Dietetics*, 4(1), 19–23.

Hawking, S. (n. d.). *Publications*. Retrieved from http://hawking.org.uk/publications.html.

Hillson, M. (2013). N. t.. In Wells, V., Wyness, L., & Coe, S. (Eds.). The British Nutrition Foundation's 45th anniversary conference: behaviour change in relation to healthier lifestyles. *Nutrition Bulletin*, 38(1), 100-107.

Hoekstra, J. H., van Kempen, A. A. M. W., & Kneepkens, C. M. F. (1993). Apple juice malabsorption: fruktose or sorbitol?. *Journal of Pediatric Gastroenterology and Nutrition*, 16(1), 39-42.

Huether, G. (Lecturer) (2014). *Interview mit Prof. Dr. Gerald Hüther zu Angst & Berufung*. Retrieved from http://www.coach-your-self.tv/Startseite/TV/InterviewmitProfDrH%c3%BctherzuAngstBerufung/tabid/1341/Default.aspx

Hyams, J. S. (1983). Sorbitol intolerance: an unappreciated cause of functional gastrointestinal complaints. *Gastroenterology*, 84(1)1, 30-33.

Hyams, J. S., Etienne, N. L., Leichtner, A. M., & Theuer, R. C. (1988). Carbohydrate malabsorption following fruit juice ingestion in young children. *Pediatrics*, 82(1), 64-68.

**Itzkowitz, S. H. & Daniel, H.** (2005). Concensus Coference: colorectal cancer screening and surveillance in inflammatory bowel disease. *Inflammatory Bowel Disease*, 11(3).

**Jameson, S.** (2000). Coeliac disease, insulin-like growth factor, bone mineral density, and zinc. *Scandinavian Journal of Gastroenterology*, 35(8), 894-896.

**Jemal, A., Siegel, R., Ward, E., Murray, T., Xu, J. Smigal, C., & Thun, M. J.** (2006). Cancer statistics, 2006. *CA: A Cancer Journal for Clinicians*, 56(2), 106-130.

**Jensen, R. G., Blanc, B., & Patton, S.** (1995). Particulate constituents in human and bovine milks. In Jensen, R. G. (Ed.), *Handbook of Milk Composition* (pp. 51-62). San Diego: Academic Press.

**Kennedy, E.** (2004). Dietary diversity, diet quality, and body weight regulation. *Nutrition Reviews*, 62(s2), S78-S81.

**Kneepkens, C. M. F., Vonk, R. J., & Fernandes, J.** (1984). Incomplete intestinal absorption of fruktose. *Archives of Disease in Childhood*, 59(8), 735-738.

**Kneepkens, C. M. F., Jakobs, C., & Douwes, A. C.** (1989): Apple juice, fruktose, and chronic nonspecific diarrhoea. *Pediatrics*, 148(6), 571-573.

**Knudsen, B. K., & Hessov, I.** (1995). Recovery of inulin from Jerusalem artichoke (Helianthus tuberosus L.) in the small intestine of man. *British Journal of Nutrition*, 74(01), 101-113.

**Komericki, P., Akkilic-Materna, M., Strimitzer, T., Weyermair, K., Hammer, H. F., & Aberer, W.** (2012). Oral xylose isomerase decreases breath hydrogen excretion and improves gastrointestinal symptoms in fruktose malabsorption – a double-blind, placebo-controlled study. *Alimentary Pharmacology & Therapeutics*, 36(10), 980-987.

**Kornbluth, A., & Sachar, D. B.** (2004). Ulcerative colitis practice guidelines in adults (update): American College of Gastroenterology, Practice Parameters Committee. *The American Journal of Gastroenterology*, 99(7), 1371-1385.

**Kuhn, R., & Gauhe, A.** (1965). Bestimmung der bindungsstelle von sialinsäureresten in oligosacchariden mit hilfe von perjodat. *Chemische Berichte*, 98(2), 395-314.

**Kupper, C.** (2005). Dietary guidelines and implementation for celiac disease. *Gastroenterology*, 128(4), 121-127.

**Kushi, L. H., Doyle, C., McCullough, M., Rock, C. L., Demark-Wahnefried, W. Bandera, E. V., ... & Gansler, T.** (2012). American cancer society guidelines on nutrition and physical activity for cancer prevention. *CA: A Cancer Journal for Clinicians*, 62(1), 30-67.

Ladas, S. D., Grammenos, I., Tassios, P. S., & Raptis, S. A. (2000). Coincidental malabsorption of laktose, fruktose, and sorbitol ingested at low doses is not Common in normal adults. *Digestive Diseases and Sciences*, 45(12), 2357-2362.

Langkilde, A. M., Andersson, H., Schweizer, T. F., & Würsch, P. (1994). Digestion and absorption of sorbitol, maltitol and isomalt from the small bowel. A study in ileostomy subjects. *European Journal of Clinical Nutrition*, 48(11), 768-775.

Latulippe, M. E., & Skoog, S. M. (2011). Fruktose malabsorption and intolerance: effects of fruktose with and without simultaneous glucose ingestion. *critical Reviews in Food Science and Nutrition*, 51(7), 583-592.

Le, A. S., & Mulderrig, K. B. (2001). *Sorbitol and Mannitol*. Nabors, O'B. (Ed.). New York, NY: Marcel Dekker.

Ledochowski, M., Sperner-Unterweger, B., Widner, B., & Fuchs, D. (1998a). Fruktose malabsorption is associated with early signs of mentral depression. *European Journal of Medical Research*, 3(6), 295-298.

Ledochowski, M., Sperner-Unterweger, B., & Fuchs, D. (1998b). Laktose malabsorption is associated with early signs of mental depression in females – a preliminary report. *Digestive Diseases and Sciences*, 43(11), 2513-2517.

Ledochowski, M., Überall, F., Propst, T., & Fuchs, D. (1999). Fruktose malabsorption is associated with lower plasma folic acid concentrations in middle-aged subjects. *Clinical Chemistry*, 45(11), 2013-2014.

Ledochowski, M., Widner, B., Bair, H., Probst, T., & Fuchs, D. (2000a). Fruktose-and sorbitol-reduced diet improves mood and gastrointestinal disturbances in fruktose malabsorbers. *Scandinavian Journal of Gastroenterology*, 35(10), 1048-1052.

Ledochowski, M., Widner, B., Sperner-Unterweger, B., Probst, T., Vogel, W., & Fuchs, D. (2000b). Carbohydrate malabsobtion syndromes and early signs of mental depression in females. *Digestive Diseases and Sciences*, 45(12), 1255-1259. [Anm. d. Verf.: Die Studie ist für Männer nicht aussagekräftig, da die Stichprobengröße zu klein ist.]

Leinoel (n. d.). *Leinöl(Leinsamen)*. Retrieved from http://www.vitalstoff-journal.de/vitalstoff-lexikon/l/leinoel-leinsamen.

Lewis, S. J., & Heaton, K. W. (1997). Stool form scale as a useful guide to intestinal transit time. *Scandinavian Journal of Gastroenterology*, 32(9), 920-924.

Lifschitz, C. H. (2000). Carbohydrate absorption from fruit juices in infants. *Pediatrics*, 105(1), e4.

Lombardi, D. A., Jin, K., Courtney, T. K., Arlinghaus, A., Folkard, S., Liang, Y., & Perry, M. J. (2014). The effects of rest breaks, work shift start time, and sleep on the onset of severe injury among workers in the People's Republic of China. *Scandinavian Journal of Work, Environment & Health*, 40(2), 146-155.

Lomer, M. C. E., Parkes, G. C., & Sanderson, J. D. (2008). Review article: Laktose intolerance in clinical practice – myths and realities. *Alimentary Pharmacology & Therapeutics*, 27(2), 93-103.

Longstreth, G. F., Thompson, W. G., chey, W. D., Houghton, L. A., Mearin, F., & Spiller, R. C. (2006). Functional bowel disorders. *Gastroenterology*, 130(5), 1480-1491.

Maintz, L., & Novak, N. (2007). Histamine and histamine intolerance. *The American Journal of Clinical Nutrition*, 85(5), 1185-1196.

Makras, L., Van Acker, G., & De Vuyst, L. (2005). Lactobacillus paracasei subsp. paracasei 8700: 2 degrades inulin-type fructans exhibiting different degrees of polymerization. *Applied and Environmental Microbiology*, 71(11), 6531-6537.

Mccoubrey, H., Parkes, G. C., Sanderson, J. D., & Lomer, M. C. E. (2008). Nutritional intakes in irritable bowel syndrome. *Journal of Human Nutrition and Dietetics*, 21(4), 396-397.

McKenzie, Y. A., Alder, A., Anderson, W. Goddard, L, Gulia, P., Jankovich, E. ...Lomer, M. C. E. (2012). British dietic association evidence-based guidelines for the dietary management of irritable bowel syndrome in adults. *Journal of Human Nutrition and Dietics*, 25(3), 260-274.

Meyrand, M., Dallas, D. C., caillat, H., Bouvier, F., Martin, P., & Barile, D. (2013). Comparison of milk oligosaccharides between goats with and without the genetic ability to synthesize αs1-casein. *Small Ruminant Research*, 113(2), 411-420.

Michel, G., Nyval-Collen, P., Barbeyron, T., czjzek, M., & Helbert, W. (2006). Bioconversion of red seaweed galactans: a focus on bacterial agarases and Carrageenases. *Applied Microbiology and Biotechnology*, 71(1), 23-33.

Michie, S. (2013). N. t.. In Wells, V., Wyness, L., & Coe, S. (Eds.). The British Nutrition Foundation's 45th anniversary conference: Behaviour change in relation to healthier lifestyles. *Nutrition Bulletin*, 38(1), 100-107.

Mishkin, D., Sablauskas, L., Yalovsky, M., & Mishkin, S. (1997). Fruktose and sorbitol malabsorption in ambulatory patients with functional dyspepsia: comparison with laktose maldigestion/malabsorption. *Digestive Diseases and Sciences*, 42(12), 2591-2598.

**Molodecky N. A., Soon, I. S., Rabi, D. M., et al.** (2012). Increasing incidence and precalence of the inflammatory bowel diseases with time, based on systematic review. *Gastroenterology,* 142(1), 46-54.

**Monash University** (2014). *The Monash University Low Foodmap Diet* [Software]. Available from http://www.med.monash.edu/cecs/gastro/fodmap/ education.html

**Montalto, M., Curigliano, V., Santoro, L., Vastola, M., Cammarota, G., Manna, R., ... & Gasbarrini, G.** (2006). Management and treatment of laktose malabsorption. *World Journal of Gastroenterology,* 12(2), 187.

**Molis, C., Flourié, B., Ouarne, F., Gailing, M. F., Lartigue, S., Guibert, A., Bornet, F., & Galmiche, F. P.** (1996). Digestion, excretion, and energy value of fructooligosaccharides in healthy humans.*The American Society for Clinical Nutrition,* 64(3), 324-328.

*Mosby's Medical Dictionary* (8th ed.). St. Louis, MO: Mosby.

**Moshfegh, A. J., James, E. F., Goldman, J. P., & Ahuja, J. L. C.** (1999). Presence of inulin and oligofruktose in the diets of Americans. *The Journal of Nutrition,* 129(7), 1407S-1411S.

**Mount Sinai** (n. d.). *Fiber Chart.* Retrieved from https://www.wehealny .org/healthinfo/dietaryfiber/fibercontentchart.html.

**Mozaffarian, D., & Wu, J. H.** (2011). Omega-3 fatty acids and cardiovascular disease effects on risk factors, molecular pathways, and clinical events. *Journal of the American College of Cardiology,* 58(20), 2047-2067.

**Muir, J. G., Shepherd, S. J., Rosella, O., Rose, R., Barrett, J. S., & Gibson, P. R.** (2007). Fructan and free fruktose content of common Australian vegetables and fruit. *Journal of Agricultural and Food Chemistry,* 55(16), 6619-6627.

**Muir, J. G., Rose, R., Rosella, O., Liels, K., Barrett, J. S., Shepherd, S. J., & Gibson, P. R.** (2009). Measurement of short-chain carbohydrates in common Australian vegetables and fruits by high-performance liquid chromatography (HPLC). *Journal of Agricultural and Food Chemistry,* 57(2), 554-565.

**Nanda, R., James, R., Smith, H., Dudley, C. R. K., & Jewell, D. P.** (1989). Food intolerance and the irritable bowel syndrome. *Gut,* 30(8), 1099-1104.

**National Digestive Diseases Information Clearinghouse** (2014). Crohn's disease. *NIH Publication,* 14-3410.

**National Digestive Diseases Information Clearinghouse** (2014). Diverticular disease. *NIH Publication,* 13-1163.

**National Digestive Diseases Information Clearinghouse** (2014). Ulcerative colitis. *NIH Publication,* 14-1597.

**Necas, J., Bartosikova, L.** (2013). Carageenan: a review. *Veterinarni Medicina,* 58(4), 187-205.

Nelis, G. F., Vermeeren, M. A., & Jansen, W. (1990). Role of fruktose-sorbitol malabsorbtion in the irritable bowel syndrome. *Gastroenterology*, 99(4), 1016-1020.

Newburg, D. S. & Neubauer, S. H. (1995). Carbohydrates in milks: analysis, quantities, and significance. In Jensen, R. G. (Ed.), *Handbook of Milk Composition* (pp. 273-349). San Diego: Academic Press.

NICNAS (2008). Multiple chemical sensitivity: identifying key research needs. *Scientific Review Report*.

Nucera, G., Gabrielli, M., Lupascu, A., Lauritano, E. C., Santoliquido, A., cremonini, F., …Gasbarrini, A. (2005). Abnormal breath tests to laktose, fruktose and sorbitol in irritable bowel syndrome may be explained by small intestinal bacterial overgrowth. *Alimentary Pharmacology & Therapeutics*, 21(11), 1391-1395.

O'Connell, J. B., Maggard, M. A., & Ko, C. Y. (2004). Colon cancer survival rates with the new American Joint Committee on Cancer sixth edition staging. *Journal of the National Cancer Institute*, 96(19), 1420-1425.

O'Connell, S., & Walsh, G. (2006). Physicochemical characteristics of commercial lactases relevant to their application in the alleviation of lactose intolerance. *Applied Biochemistry and Biotechnology*, 134(2), 179-191.

Ong, D., Mitchell, S., Barrett, J., Shepherd, S., Irving, P., Biesiekierski, J., & … Muir, J. (2010). Manipulation of dietary short chain carbohydrates alters the pattern of gas production and genesis of symptoms in irritable bowel syndrome. *Journal of Gastroenterology & Hepatology*, 25(8), 1366-1373.

Park, Y. K., & Yetley, E. A. (1993). Intakes and food sources of fruktose in the United States. *The American Journal of Clinical Nutrition*, 58(5), 737S-747S.

Parker, T. J., Naylor, S. J., Riordan, A. M., & Hunter, J. O. (1995). Management of patients with food intolerance in irritable bowel syndrome. The development and use of an exclusion diet. *Journal of Human Nutrition and Dietetics*, 8(3), 159-166.

Peery, A. F., Barrett, P. R. Park, D., et al. (2012). A high-fiber diet does not protect against asymptomatic diverticulosis. *Gastroenterology*, 142(2), 266-272.

Petitpierre, M., Gumowski, P., & Girard, J. P. (1985). Irritable bowel syndrome and hypersensitivity to food. *Annals of Allergy, Asthma & Immunology*, 54(6), 538-540.

Quigley, E., Fried, M., Gwee, K. A., Olano, C., Guarner, F., Khalif, I., … & Le Mair, A. W. (2009). Irritable bowel syndrome: a global perspective. *WGO Practice Guideline*.

Quigley, E., M., M., Hunt, R. H., Emmanuel, A., & Hungin, A. P. S. (2013). *Irritable bowel syndrome (ibs): what is it, what causes it and can i do anything about it?* Retrieved from http://client.blueskybroadcastcom/WGO/ index.html.

Raithel, M., Weidenhiller, M., Hagel, A.-F.-K., Hetterich, U., Neurath, M. F., & Konturek, P. C. (2013). The malabsorption of commonly occurring mono and disaccharides: levels of investigation and differential diagnoses. *Dtsch Arztebl Int*, 110(46), 775-782.

Rex, D. K., Johnson, D. A., Anderson, J. C., Schoenfeld, P. S., Burke, C. A., & Inadomi, J. M. (2009). American College of Gastroenterology guidelines for colorectal cancer screening 2008. *The American Journal of Gastroenterology*, 104(3), 739-750.

Riby, J. E., Fujisawa, T., & Kretchmer, N. (1993). Fruktose absorption. *The American Journal of Clinical Nutrition*, 58(5), 748S-753S.

Ross, A. C., Manson, J. E., Abrams, S. A., Aloia, J. F., Brannon, P. M., Clinton, S. K., ... & Shapses, S. A. (2011). The 2011 report on dietary reference intakes for calcium and vitamin D from the Institute of Medicine: what clinicians need to know. *Journal of Clinical Endocrinology & Metabolism*, 96(1), 53-58.

Rubio-Tapia, A., Hill, I. D., Kelly, C. P., Calderwood, A. H., & Murray, J. A. (2013). ACG clinical guidelines: diagnosis and management of celiac disease.*The American Journal of Gastroenterology*, 108(5), 656-676.

Rumessen, J. J., & Gudmand-Høyer, E. (1986). Absorption capacity of fruktose in healthy adults. comparison with sucrose and its constituent monosaccharides. *Gut*, 27(10), 1161-1168.

Rumessen, J. J., & Gudmand-Høyer, E. (1987). Malabsoption of fruktose-sorbitol mixtures. Interactions causing abdominal distress. *Scandinavian Journal of Gastroenterology*, 22(4), 431-436.

Rumessen, J. J. (1992). Fruktose and related food carbohydrates. sources, intake, absorbtion, and clinical implications. *Scandinavian Journal of Gastroenterology*, 27(10), 819-828.

Ruppin, H., Bar-Meir, S., Soergel, K. H., Wood, C. M., & Schmitt Jr, M. G. (1980). Absorption of short-chain fatty acids by the colon. *Gastroenterology*, 78(6), 1500-1507.

Rycroft, C. E., Jones, M. R., Gibson, G. R., & Rastall, R. A. (2001). A comparative in vitro evaluation of the fermentation properties of prebiotic oligosaccharides. *Journal of Applied Microbiology*, 91(5), 878-887.

Scientific Community on Food (2000). *Opinion of the Scientific Committee on Food on the tolerable upper intake level of folate.* Retrieved from: www.ec.europa.eu/food/fc/sc/scf/out80e_en.pdf

**Shepherd, S. J., & Gibson, P. R.** (2006). Fruktose malabsorption and symptoms of irritable bowel syndrome: guidelines for effective dietary management. *Journal of the American Dietetic Association*, 106(10), 1631-1639.

**Shepherd, S. J., Parker, F. C., Muir, J. G., & Gibson, P. R.** (2008). Dietary triggers of abdominal symptoms in patients with irritable bowel syndrome: randomized placebo-controlled evidence. *Clinical Gastroenterology and Hepatology*, 6(7), 765-771.

**Silk, D. B. A., Davis, A., Vulevic, J., Tzortzis, G., & Gibson, G. R.** (2009). Clinical trial: the effects of a trans-galactooligosaccharide prebiotic on faecal microbiota and symptoms in irritable bowel syndrome. *Alimentary Pharmacology & Therapeutics*, 29(5), 508-518.

**Simopoulos, A. P.** (1999). Essential fatty acids in health and chronic disease. *The American Journal of Clinical Nutrition*, 70(3), 560s-569s.

**Speier, C., Vessey, I., & Valacich, J. S.** (2003). The effects of interruptions, task complexity, and information presentation on computer-supported decision-making performance. *Decision Sciences*, 34(4), 771-797.

**Stefanini, G. F., Saggioro, A., Alvisi, V., Angelini, G., capurso, L., Di, L. G., ...Melzi, G.** (1995). Oral cromolyn sodium in comparison with elimination diet in the irritable bowel syndrome, diarrheic type. multicenter study of 428 patients. *Scandinavian Journal of Gastroenterology*, 30(6), 535–541.

**Stockwell, M.** (n. d.). *Awards/Events*. Retrieved from www.melissastock well.com/Melissa_Stockwell/Awards.html.

**Stubbs, J.** (2013). N. t.. In Wells, V., Wyness, L., & Coe, S. (Eds.). The British Nutrition Foundation's 45th anniversary conference: behaviour change in relation to healthier lifestyles. *Nutrition Bulletin*, 38(1), 100-107.

**Suarez, F. L., Savaiano, D. A., & Levitt, M. D.** (1995). A comparison of symptoms after the consumption of milk or laktose-hydrolyzed milk by people with self-reported severe laktose intolerance. *New England Journal of Medicine*, 333(1), 1-4.

**Suarez, F. L., Springfield, J., Furne, J. K., Lohrmann, T. T., Kerr, P. S., & Levitt, M. D.** (1999). Gas production in humans ingesting a soybean flour derived from beans naturally low in oligosaccharides. *The American Journal of Clinical Nutrition*, 69(1), 135-139.

**Sundhedsstyrelsen og Fødevareministeriet** (2009). *Cøliaki og mad uden Gluten* (4th ed.). København: Sundhedsstyrelsen.

**Tarpila, S., Tarpila, A., Grohn, P., Silvennoinen, T., & Lindberg, L.** (2004). Efficacy of ground flaxseed on constipation in patients with irritable bowel syndrome. *Current Topics in Nutraceutical Research*, 2(2), 119–125.

Test (2008). Schneller, schöner, stärker. *test – Journal Gesundheit*, 43(02), 88-92.

Teuri, U., Vapaatalo, H., & Korpela, R. (1999). Fructooligosaccharides and lactulose cause more symptoms in laktose maldigesters and subjects with pseudohypolactasia than in control laktose digesters. *The American Journal of Clinical Nutrition*, 69(5), 973-979.

Thompson, Kyle (2006). *Bristol Stool Chart* [Graphical illustration]. Retrieved from http://commons.wikimedia.org/wiki/File:Bristol_Stool_chart.png

Nanda, R., Shu, L. H., & Thomas, J. R. (2012). A fodmap diet update: craze or credible. *Practical Gastroenterology*, 10(12), 37-46.

Toschke, A. M., Thorsteinsdottir, K. H., & von Kries, R. (2009). Meal frequency, breakfast consumption and childhood obesity. *International Journal of Pediatric Obesity*, 4(4), 242-248.

Tou, J. C., Chen, J., & Thompson, L. U. (1998). Flaxseed and its lignan precursor, secoisolariciresinol diglycoside, affect pregnancy outcome and reproductive development in rats. *The Journal of Nutrition*, 128(11), 1861-1868.

Truswell, A. S., Seach, J. M., & Thorburn, A. W. (1988). Incomplete absorption of pure fruktose in healthy subjects and the facilitating effect of glucose. *The American Journal of Clinical Nutrition*, 48(6), 1424-1430.

U. S. Department of Agriculture and U. S. Department of Health and Human Services (2010). *Dietary Guidelines for Americans* (7th ed.). Washington, Dc: U. S. Government Printing Office.

U. S. Department of Agriculture, Agricultural Research Service (2013). *USDA National Nutrient Database for Standard Reference*, Release 26. Retrieved from: http://www.ars.usda.gov/ba/bhnrc /ndl.

van Loo, J., Coussement, P., De Leenheer, L., Hoebregs, H., & Smits, G. (1995). On the presence of inulin and oligofruktose as natural ingredients in the western diet. *Critical Reviews in Food Science and Nutrition*, 35(6), 525–552.

Varea, V., de Carpi, J. M., Puig, C., Alda, J. A., camacho, E., Ormazabal, A., ... & Gómez, L. (2005). Malabsorption of carbohydrates and depression in Children and adolescents. *Journal of Pediatric Gastroenterology and Nutrition*, 40(5), 561-565.

Verhoef, P., Stampfer, M. J., Buring, J. F., Gaziano, J. M., Allen, R. H., Stabler, S. P., ... & Willett, W. C. (1996). Homocysteine metabolism and risk of myocardial infarction: relation with vitamins B6, B12, and folate. *American Journal of Epidemiology*, 143(9), 845-859.

Vernia, P., Ricciardi, M. R., Frandina, C., Bilotta, T., & Frieri, G. (1995). laktose malabsorption and irritable bowel syndrome. Effect of a long-term laktose-free diet. *The Italian Journal of Gastroenterology*, 27(3), 117-121.

**Vesa, T. H., Korpela, R. A., & Sahi, T.** (1996). Tolerance to small amounts of laktose in laktose maldigesters. *The AmericanJournal of Clinical Nutrition, 64*(2), 197-20.

**Virtanen, S. M., Räsänen, L., Mäenpää, J., & Åkerblom, H. K.** (1987). Dietary survey of Finnish adolescent diabetics and non-diabetic controls. *Acta Paediatrica, 76*(5), 801-808.

**Vos, M. B., Kimmons, J. E., Gillespie, C., Welsh, J., & Blanck, H. M.** (2008). Dietary fruktose consumption among US children and adults: the third National Health and Nutrition Examination Survey. *The Medscape Journal of Medicine, 10*(7), 160.

**Watson, B. D.** (2008). Public health and carrageenan regulation : a review and analysis. *Journal of Applied Phycology, 20*(5), 505-513.

**Webb, F. S., & Whitney, E. N.** (2008). *Nutrition: Concepts and Controversies* (11th ed.). Belmont, CA: Thomson/ Wadsworth.

**Wedlake, L., Slack, N., Andreyev, H. J. N., & Whelan, K.** (2014). Fiber in the treatment and maintenance of inflammatory bowel disease: a systematic review of randomized controlled trials. *Inflammatory bowel diseases, 20*(3), 576-586.

**Welch, C. E., Allen, A. W., & Donaldons, G. A.** (1953). An appraisal of resection of the colon for diverticulitis of the sigmoid. *Annals of Surgery, 138*(3), 332-343.

**Wells, N. E. J., Hahn, B. A., & Whorwell, P. J.** (1997). Clinical economics review: irritable bowel syndrome. *Allimentary Pharmacology and Therapeutics, 11*, 1019-1030.

—

**Sources regarding the prevalence of IBS:**
**Great Britain**

**Jones, R., & Lydeard, S.** (1992). Irritable bowel syndrom in the general population. *British Medical Journal, 304*(6819), 87-90.

**Japan and the Netherlands**

**Schlemper, R. J., van der Werf, S. D. J., Vandenbroucke, J. P., Blemond, I., & Lamers, C. B. H. W.** (1993). Peptic ulcer, non-ulcer dysepsia and irritable bowel syndrom in the Netherlands and Japan. *Scandinavian Journal of Gastroenterology, 28*(200), 33-41.

**Nigeria**

**Olubuykle, I. O., Olawuyl, F., & Fasanmade, A. A.** (1995). A study of irritable bowel syndrom diagnosed by manning Criteria in an African population. *Digestive Diseases and Sciences, 40*(5), 983-985.

**USA**

Longstreth, G. F., & Wolde-Tsadik, G. (1993). Irritable bowel-type symptoms in hmo examinees. *Digestive Diseases and Sciences*, 38(9), 1581-1589.

Talley, N. J., Zinsmeister, A. R., van Dyke, C., & Melton, L. J. (1991). Epidemiology of colonic symptoms and the irritable bowel syndrome. *Gastroenterology*, 101(4), 927-934.

O'Keefe, E. A., Talley, N. J., Zinsmeister, A. R., & Jacobsen, S. J. (1995). Bowel disorders impair functional status and quality of life in the elerdly: a population-based study. *Journal of Gastroenterology*, 50A, M184-M189.

—

Wilder-Smith, C. H., Materna, A., Wermelinger, C., & Schuler, J. (2013). Fruktose and laktose intolerance and malabsorption testing: the relationship with symptoms in functional gastrointestinal disorders. *Alimentary Pharmacology and Therapeutics*, 37(11), 1074-1083.

Winterfeldt, D. von, & Edwards, W. (1986). *Decision Analysis and Behavioral Research*. Cambridge: Cambridge University Press.

Wittstock, A. (1949). *Marc Aurel – Selbstbetrachtungen*. Stuttgart: Reclam.

Zohar, D. (1999). When things go wrong: The effect of daily work hassles on effort, exertion and negative mood. *Journal of Occupational and Organizational Psychology*, 72(3), 265-283.

# Food Index

Basmati rice, cooked in unsalted water 146

BBQ roasted jalapeno sauce 148

Beef bacon (kosher) 142

Beef steak, chuck, visible fat eaten 142

Beef with noodles soup, condensed 137

Beer 95

Beer, low alcohol 95

Beer, low carb 95

Beer, non alcoholic 95

Beets, raw 162

Ben & Jerry's® Ice Cream, Brownie Batter 169

Ben & Jerry's® Ice Cream, Chocolate Chip Cookie Dough 169

Ben & Jerry's® Ice Cream, Chubby Hubby® 169

Ben & Jerry's® Ice Cream, Chunky Monkey® 169

Ben & Jerry's® Ice Cream, Half Baked 169

Ben & Jerry's® Ice Cream, Karamel Sutra® 169

Ben & Jerry's® Ice Cream, New York Super Fudge Chunk® 169

Ben & Jerry's® Ice Cream, One Sweet Whirled 169

Ben & Jerry's® Ice Cream, Peanut Butter Cup 169

Ben & Jerry's® Ice Cream, Phish Food® 169

Ben & Jerry's® Ice Cream, Vanilla For A Change 169

Biscotti, chocolate, nuts 128

BK Big Fish® 148

BK Fresh Apple Slices 148

Black beans, cooked from dried 162

Black cherry juice 105

Black currant juice 105

Black olives 162

Black Russian 95

Blackberries, fresh 157

Blackberry juice 105

Bloody Mary 95

BLT Salad® with TenderCrisp chicken (no dressing or croutons) 148

Blue cheese 116

Blueberries, fresh 157

Bockwurst 142

Bok choy, raw 162

Bologna, beef ring 116

Bologna, combination of meats, light (reduced fat) 116

Boston Market® 1/4 white rotisserie chicken, with skin 142

Boston Market® macaroni and cheese 137

Boston Market® roasted turkey breast 142

Boston Market® sweet corn 146

Bourbon 95

Boysenberries, fresh 157

Brandy 95

Bratwurst 142

Bratwurst, beef 142

Bratwurst, light (reduced fat) 142

Bratwurst, made with beer 142

Bratwurst, made with beer, cheese-filled 142

Bratwurst, turkey 142

Braunschweiger 142

Brazil nuts, unsalted 125

Breath mint, regular 133

Breath mint, sugar free 133

Breyers® Ice Cream, Natural Vanilla, Lactose Free 169

Breyers® Light! Boosts Immunity Yogurt, all flavors 120

Breyers® No Sugar Added Ice Cream, Vanilla 120

Breyers® YoCrunch Light Nonfat Yogurt, with granola 120

Cherry pie, bottom crust only 128
Chestnuts, boiled, steamed 163
Chestnuts, roasted 125
Chewing gum 133
Chewing gum, sugar free 133
Chia seeds 125
Chicken and dumplings soup, condensed 137
Chicken breast, spicy crispy 150
Chicken cake or patty 145
Chicken fricassee with gravy, American style 142
Chicken Littles with sauce 150
Chicken noodle soup with vegetables, can 137
Chicken with cheese sauce, vegetables other than dark green 145
Chicken wonton soup, prepared from condensed can 137

Chicory coffee 101
Chicory coffee powder, unprepared 163
Chicory greens, raw 163
Chili with beans, beef, canned 137
Chipotle southwest salad dressing 153
Chips Ahoy!® Chewy Gooey Caramel Cookies (Nabisco®) 128
Chobani® Nonfat Greek Yogurt, Black Cherry 120
Chobani® Nonfat Greek Yogurt, Lemon 120
Chobani® Nonfat Greek Yogurt, Peach 120
Chobani® Nonfat Greek Yogurt, Raspberry 120
Chobani® Nonfat Greek Yogurt, Strawberry 120
Chocolate cake, glazed, store 128
Chocolate Chex® (General Mills®) 113
Chocolate chip cookie 153

Chocolate chip cookies, store bought 129
Chocolate chunk cookie 153
Chocolate cookies, iced, store bought 129
Chocolate pudding, store bought 120
Chocolate pudding, store bought, no sugar 120
Chocolate sandwich cookies, double filling 129
Chocolate sandwich cookies, sugar free 129
Chocolate truffles 133
Chop suey, chicken 138
Chop suey, tofu, no noodles 138
Cinnamon crispas 129
Cinnamon toast crunch® (General Mills®) 113
Cinnamon Toasters® (Malt-O-Meal®) 113
Clams, with mushroom, onions, & bread 142

Classic Fruit Chocolates (Liberty Orchards®) 133
Clementine, fresh 157
Clif Bar®,Chocolate Chip 93
Clif Bar®,Crunchy Peanut Butter 93
Clif Bar®,Oatmeal Raisin Walnut 93
Club soda 96
Cocoa Krispies® (Kellogg's®) 113
Cocoa Puffs® (General Mills®) 113
Coconut Bars, nuts 133
Coconut cream (liquid from grated meat) 125
Coconut milk, fresh (liquid from grated meat, water added) 125
Coconut, dried, shredded or flaked, unsweetened 125
Coconut, fresh 125
Coffee substitute, prepared 101

Coffee, prepared from flavored mix, no sugar 101
Cognac 96
Cointreau® 96
Coke Zero® 108
Coke® 108
Coke® with Lime 108
Colby Jack cheese 116
Cole slaw 150
Coleslaw, with apples and raisins, mayo dressing 163
Coleslaw, with pineapple, mayo dressing 163
Collards, raw 163
Corn Chex® (General Mills®) 113
Corn Flakes (Kellogg's®) 113
Cornbread, from mix 146
Cornbread, homemade 146
Cottage cheese, 1% fat, lactose reduced 116
Cottage cheese, uncreamed dry curd 120
Couscous, cooked 146

Cracked wheat bread, with raisins 111
Cranberries, dried (Craisins®) 158
Cranberries, fresh 158
Cranberry juice cocktail, with apple juice 105
Cranberry juice cocktail, with blueberry juice 105
Cream cheese spread 117
Cream cheese, whipped, flavored 117
Cream cheese, whipped, plain 117
Cream of asparagus soup, condensed can 138
Cream of broccoli soup, condensed 138
Cream of celery soup, homemade 138
Cream of chicken soup, condensed 138
Cream of mushroom soup, from condensed can 138

Cream of potato soup mix, dry 138
Cream of spinach soup mix, dry 138
Creamed chicken 145
Creamy buffalo sauce 150
Creme de Cocoa 96
Creme de menthe 96
Crepe, plain 129
Crispy Chicken Caesar Salad 150
Crispy Twister without sauce 150
Crispy Twister® with sauce 150
Croissant, chocolate 129
Croissant, fruit 129
Crunchy Nut Roasted Nut & Honey (Kellogg's®) 113
Cucumber, raw, with peel 164

Cucumber, raw, without peel 164
Curacao 96
Currants, fresh, black 158
Currants, fresh, red and white 158

**D**

Daiquiri 96
Dairy Queen® Foot Long Hot Dog 138
Dandelion tea 102
Danish pastry, frosted, with cheese filling 129
Dannon® Activia® Light Yogurt, vanilla 121
Dannon® Activia® Yogurt, plain 121
Dannon® Greek Yogurt Honey 121
Dannon® Greek Yogurt, Plain 121
Dannon® la Crème Yogurt, fruit flavors 121
Dare Breaktime Ginger Cookies 129
Dare® Lemon Crème Cookies 129
Dark chocolate Bar 50% 133
Dark chocolate Bar 60%-69% cacao 134
Dark chocolate Bar 70%-85% cacao 134

Dark chocolate Bar, sugar free 134

Dark Fruit Chocolates (Liberty Orchards®) 134

Dark Fruit Chocolates, Sugar Free (Liberty Orchards®) 134

Dates 158

Demitasse 102

Diet 7 UP® 108

Diet Coke® 108

Diet Dr. Pepper® 108

Diet Pepsi®, fountain 108

Doritos® Tortilla Chips, Nacho Cheese 125

Doughnut, glazed, coconut topping 129

Doughnut, glazed, plain 129

Doughnut, sugared 129

Dove® Promises, Milk Chocolate 102

Dreyer's® Grand Ice Cream, Chocolate 169

Dreyer's® No Sugar Added Ice Cream, Triple Chocolate 169

Drumstick® (sundae cone) 170

**E**

Earl Grey, strong 102

Edam cheese 117

EGG® bread roll 129

Eggnog, regular 96

Eggplant, cooked 164

Elderberries, fresh 158

Electrolyte drink 93

Elephant ear (crispy) 129

Endive, curly, raw 164

English muffin bread 111

English muffin, whole wheat, with raisins 130

Enoki mushrooms, raw 164

Espresso, raw 102

Essentials Oat Bran cereal (Quaker®) 113

Evaporated milk, diluted, 2% fat (reduced fat) 121

Evaporated milk, skim (fat free) 102

Evaporated milk, whole 121

Extra Crispy Tenders 150

**F**

Falafel 146

Familia Swiss Muesli® 113

Fanta Zero®, fruit flavors 108

Fanta® Red 108

Fanta®, fruit flavors 108

Fennel bulb 164

Fennel tea 102

Feta cheese 121

Feta cheese, fat free 121

Fettuccini Alfredo®, no meat, carrots or dark green veggies 138

Fettuccini Alfredo®, no meat, vegetables except dark green 138

Fettuccini noodles 146

Fiber One Original® (General Mills®) 114

Fiber One® Nutty Clusters & Almonds (General Mills®) 114

Fifty 50® Sugar Free Butterscotch Hard Candy 134

Figs, dried, cooked, sweetened 158

Figs, fresh 158

Filberts, raw 125

Fish croquette 145

Fish or seafood with cream or white sauce 145

Fish sticks, patties / nuggets, breaded, 143

Fish with breading 143

Flax seeds, not fortified 125

Fleischmann's® Butter Margarine, tub, whipped 117

Focaccia bread 111

Fondue sauce 121

Frappuccino® 102

Frappuccino®, bottled or canned 102

Frappuccino®, bottled light 102

French Burnt Peanuts 134

French fries 148

French or Vienna roll 111

French toast 130

Froot Loops® (Kellogg's®) 114

Frosted Flakes®
(Kellogg's®) 114
Frosted Flakes®
Reduced Sugar
(Kellogg's®) 114
Frosted Mini-
Wheats Big Bite®
(Kellogg's®) 114
Frozen custard,
chocolate or cof-
fee flavors 130
Frozen fruit juice
Bar 170
Fruit drink or
punch 105
Fruit punch, alco-
holic 96
Fruit sauce, jelly-
based 138

**G**
Garbanzo beans
canned 146
Garlic, fresh 164
Gatorade®, all fla-
vors 93
Gelatin, jello 134
German choco-
late cake, glazed,
homemade 130
German style po-
tato salad, with
bacon and vine-
gar dressing 138
GG® Scandina-
vian Bran Crisp-
bread 111

Gibson 97
Gin 97
Ginger ale 108
Ginger root, raw
164
Ginko nuts, dried
126
Girl Scout® Lem-
onades 130
Girl Scout® Pea-
nut Butter Patties
130
Girl Scout® Sa-
moas® 130
Girl Scout® Short-
bread® 130
Girl Scout® Thin
Mints 130
Glaceau® Vita-
minwater 93
Gluten free bread
111
GO Veggie!™
Rice Slices 121
Goat cheese, hard
117
GoLEAN® Crisp!
Cereal, Cinna-
mon Crumble
(Kashi®) 114
GoLEAN®
Crunch! Cereal,
Honey Almond
Flax (Kashi®) 114
Gooseberries,
fresh 158
Gorgonzola
cheese 117

Gorton's® Bat-
tered Fish Fillets
143
Gorton's® Pop-
corn Shrimp,
Original 143
Gouda cheese 117
Goulash, with
beef, noodles, to-
mato base 143
Grand Marnier®
97
Grapefruit juice,
white 105
Grapefruit, fresh,
pink or red 158
Grapes, fresh 158
Grasshopper 97
Greek yogurt,
plain, nonfat, 121
Green beans
(string beans),
cooked 164
Green bell pep-
pers 164
Green olives 164
Green pea soup
138
Green peas, raw
146
Green tea, strong
102
Green tomato,
raw 164
Grits (polenta)
164
Guava (guayaba),
fresh, 158

Gum drops 134
Gum drops,
sugar free 134
Gummi bears 134
Gummi bears,
sugar free 134
Gummi dino-
saurs 134
Gummi dino-
saurs, no sugar
134
Gummi worms
134
Gummi worms,
sugar free 135

**H**
Haagen-Dazs®
Creme Brulee 170
Haagen-Dazs®
Frozen Yogurt,
chocolate or cof-
fee flavors 170
Haagen-Dazs®
Frozen Yogurt,
vanilla or other
flavors 170
Haagen-Dazs® Ice
Cream, Bailey's
Irish Cream 170
Haagen-Dazs® Ice
Cream, Black
Walnut 170
Haagen-Dazs® Ice
Cream, Butter Pe-
can 170

Haagen-Dazs® Cherry Vanilla 170

Haagen-Dazs® Ice Cream, Chocolate 170

Haagen-Dazs® Ice Cream, Coffee 170

Haagen-Dazs® Ice Cream, Cookies & Cream 170

Haagen-Dazs® Ice Cream, Mango 170

Haagen-Dazs® Ice Cream, Pistachio 170

Haagen-Dazs® Ice Cream, Rocky Road 170

Haagen-Dazs® Ice Cream, Strawberry 171

Haagen-Dazs® Ice Cream, Vanilla Chocolate Chip 171

Half and half 121

Halvah 130

Ham croquette 145

Ham Sandwich with Veggies, no mayo 153

Hamburger 148

Hard candy 135

Hard candy, sugar free 135

Hardee's® Loaded Omelet Biscuit 138

Harvey Wallbanger 97

Health Valley® Multigrain Chewy Granola Bar, Chocolate Chip 114

Herbal tea 102

Herring, pickled 143

Hershey's® Bliss Hot Drink White Chocolate, prepared 102

Hershey's® Caramel Filled Chocolates no sugar 135

Hershey's® Milk Chocolate Bar 135

Hickorynuts 126

High-protein Bar, generic 93

Honey 114

Honey BBQ sauce 150

Honey mustard dressing 153

Honey Nut Chex® (General Mills®) 114

Honey Oat bread 153

Honey Smacks® (Kellogg's®) 114

Honeydew 158

Hot chili peppers, green, cooked 164

Hot chili peppers, red, cooked from fresh 164

Hot chocolate, homemade 102

Hot dog, combination of meats, plain 117

Hot wings 150

House side salad 150

Hubbard squash 165

**I**

Ice cream sandwich 171

Ice cream, light 171

Instant coffee mix, unprepared 102

Irish coffee with alcohol and whipped cream 102

Italian BMT® Sandwich with Veggies, no mayo 153

**J**

Jackfruit, fresh 158

Jam 117

Jam no sugar or sweetener 118

Jasmine tea 103

Jelly beans® 135

Jelly beans®, sugar free 135

Jerusalem artichoke raw 165

Jujyfruits® 135

**K**

Kale, raw 165

Kamikaze 97

Kashi® Chewy Granola Bar, Cherry Dark Chocolate 114

Kashi® Layered Granola Bar, Pumpkin Pecan 135

Kefir 121

Kelp, raw 165

Ken's® Apple Cider Vinaigrette dressing 148

Kern's® Mango-Orange Nectar 105

Kern's® Strawberry Nectar 105

Kidney beans, cooked from dried 165

Kirsch 97

Kit Kat® 135

Kit Kat® White 135

Kiwi fruit, gold 158

Kiwi fruit, green 158

Kohlrabi, cooked 165

Kraft® Cheese Spread, Roka Blue 118

**L**

Lasagna, homemade, beef 139

Lasagna, homemade, cheese, no vegetables 139

Lasagna, homemade, spinach, no meat 139

Laughing Cow® Mini Babybel®, Cheddar 121

Laughing Cow® Mini Babybel®, Original 122

Lay's® Potato Chips 126

Lay's® Potato Chips, Sour Cream & Onion 126

Lay's® Stax Potato Crisps, Cheddar 126

Lay's® Stax Potato Crisps, Hot 'n Spicy 126

Lebkuchen (German ginger bread) 130

Leeks, leafs 165

Leeks, root 165

Leeks, whole 165

Lemon juice, fresh 106

Lemon peel 172

Lemon, fresh 159

Lentil soup, condensed 139

Lentils, cooked from dried 146

Lettuce, Boston, bibb or butterhead 165

Lettuce, green leaf 165

Lettuce, iceberg 165

Lettuce, red leaf 165

Lettuce, romaine or cos 165

Libby's® Apricot Nectar 106

Libby's® Banana Nectar 106

Libby's® Juicy Juice®, Apple Grape 106

Libby's® Juicy Juice®, Grape 106

Libby's® Pear Nectar 106

Licorice 135

Licuado, mango 122

Light beer 97

Light cream 122

Lima beans, cooked from dried 165

Limburger cheese 118

Lime juice, fresh 106

Lime, fresh 159

Lipton® Iced Tea Mix, sweetened with sugar, prepared 109

Lipton® Instant 100% Tea, unsweetened, prepared 109

Liqueur, coffee flavored 97

Little Debbie® Coffee Cake, Apple Streusel 130

Little Debbie® Fudge Brownies with Walnuts 130

Little Debbie® Nutty Bars 135

Liver pudding 143

Loaf cold cut, spiced 145

Loganberries, fresh 159

Long Island iced tea 97

Long John or bismarck, glazed, cream or custard filled & nuts 130

Lotus root, cooked 166

Lowbush cranberries (lingonberries) 159

Lychees (litchis), fresh 159

Lycium (wolf or goji berries) 159

Lyonnaise (potatoes and onions) 139

M & M® cookie 153

M & M's® Peanut 135

Macadamia nuts, raw 126

Macaroni or pasta salad, with meat, egg, mayo dressing 139

Mai Tai 97

Maitake mushrooms, raw 166

Malt liquor 97

Mamba® Fruit Chews 135

Mamba® Sour Fruit Chews 135

**M**

Mandarin orange, fresh 159

Mango nectar 106

Mango, fresh 159

Mangosteen, fresh 159

Manhattan 97

Maple syrup, pure 114

Margarine, diet, fat free 118

Margarine, tub, salted, sunflower oil 118

Margarita, frozen 97

Marmalade, sugar free with aspartame 118

Marmalade with saccharin 118

Marmalade, sugar free with sucralose 118

Marshmallow 135

Martini® 97

Mascarpone 118

Mashed potatoes with gravy 150

McDonald's® apple slices 151

McDonald's® Barbecue sauce 151

McDonald's® Big Mac® 151

McDonald's® caramel sundae® 151

McDonald's® Cheeseburger 151

McDonald's® Chicken McNuggets® 151

McDonald's® chocolate chip cookies 151

McDonald's® chocolate milk 151

McDonald's® Crispy Chicken Snack Wrap with ranch sauce 151

McDonald's® Double Cheeseburger 151

McDonald's® Filet-O-Fish® 151

McDonald's® French fries 151

McDonald's® Hamburger 151

McDonald's® hot fudge sundae® 151

McDonald's® hot mustard 151

McDonald's® M & M McFlurry® 152

McDonald's® McCafe shakes, chocolate 152

McDonald's® McCafe shakes, vanilla or other flavors 152

McDonald's® McChicken® 152

McDonald's® McDouble® 152

McDonald's® McRib® 152

McDonald's® Newman's Own® Creamy Caesar dressing 152

McDonald's® Newman's Own® Low Fat Balsamic Vinaigrette salad dressing 152

McDonald's® orange juice 152

McDonald's® Quarter Pounder 152

McDonald's® Sausage & EGG® McMuffin® 152

McDonald's® side salad 152

McDonald's® smoothies, all flavors 152

McDonald's® Southwestern chipotle Barbecue sauce 152

McDonald's® sweet and sour sauce 152

Meat ravioli, with tomato sauce 139

Meatloaf, pork 145

Meatloaf, tuna 145

Melba Toast®, Classic (Old London®) 126

Mentos® 135

Merlot, red 97

Merlot, white 98

Milk chocolate Bar, cereal 135

Milk chocolate Bar, cereal, sugar free 135

Milk chocolate Bar, sugar free 135

Milk Chocolate covered raisins 135

Milk Maid® Caramels (Brach's®) 135

Milk, low lactose Lactaid®, skim (fat free) 122

Milk, lactose reduced Lactaid®, fortified 114

Milk, low lactose Lactaid® 103

Milk, unprepared dry powder, 103

Mineral Water 109

Minestrone soup, condensed 139

Minestrone soup, homemade 139
Mint Julep 98
Mocha, pure 103
Mojito 98
Molasses cookies, store bought 130
Molasses, dark 135
Monster® Energy® 109
Monster® Khaos 109
Morel mushrooms, raw 166
Mortadella 118
Mountain Dew® 109
Mountain Dew® Code Red 109
Mozzarella, fat free 122
Mrs. Paul's® Calamari Rings 143
Muenster cheese, natural 118
Mueslix® (Kellogg's®) 115
Muffins, banana 130
Muffins, blueberry 131
Muffins, carrot, homemade, with nuts 131
Muffins, store bought 131

Muffins, pumpkin, 131
Mulberries 159
Mung bean sprouts 166
Mung beans, cooked from dried 166
Murray® Sugar Free Oatmeal Cookies 131
Murray® Sugar Free Shortbread 131
Muscatel 98
Mushrooms, batter dipped or breaded 166
Muskmelon 159
Mustard 153

**N**
Nabisco® 100 Calorie Packs, Honey Maid Cinnamon Roll 131
Nectarine 159
Nestea® 100% Tea, dry 109
Nestea® Iced Tea, Sugar Free, dry 109
Nestea® Iced Tea, no sugar 109Nestea® Iced Tea, with sugar, dry 109

Nestle® Hot Cocoa Dark Chocolate, prepared 103
Nestle® Hot Cocoa Rich Milk Chocolate 103
Nestle® Nesquik®, chocolate dry 135
Newman's Own® Organic Pretzels 111
Nilla Wafers® (Nabisco®) 131
No Fear® 109
No Fear® Sugar Free 109
Non-alcoholic wine 98
Noodle soup mix, dry 139
Northland® Cranberry Juice, all flavors 106
Nougat 135
Nutella® (filbert spread) 118
Nutter Butter® Cookies (Nabisco®) 131

**O**
Oat milk 122
Oatmeal cookies, store bought 131
Okra, raw 166
Old Dutch® Crunch Curls 126

Omelet, made with bacon 139
Omelet, made with sausage, potatoes, onions, cheese 139
Onion rings 148
Onion, white, yellow or red, raw 166
Oolong tea 103
Orange kiwi passion juice 106
Orange peel 172
Orange, fresh 159
Oreo® Brownie Cookies 131
Oreo® Cookies (Nabisco®) 131
Oreo® Cookies, Sugar Free 131
Chicken Crisp® Sandwich 148
Ouzo 98
Oven Roasted Chicken Sandwich with Veggies, no mayo 153
Oyster mushrooms, raw 166

**P**
Pad Thai, without meat 139
Paella 139
Pancake, buckwheat 131

Pancake, whole wheat, homemade 131
Pancakes and syrup 149
Panda Express® Orange Chicken 139
Papaya, fresh 159
Parmesan cheese, dry (grated) 122
Parmesan cheese, dry (grated), non-fat 122
Parmesan Oregano bread 153
Parsnip, cooked 166
Passion fruit (maracuya), fresh 159
Passion fruit juice 106
Pasta salad with vegetables, Italian dressing 139
Peach juice 106
Peach pie, bottom crust only 131
Peach, fresh 159
Peanut butter, unsalted 126
Peanuts, dry roasted, salted 126
Pear juice 106
Pear, fresh 160
Pecan praline 135

Pepperidge Farm® Soft Sugar Cookies 132
Pepperidge Farm® Turnover, Apple 132
Pepsi® 109
Pepsi® Max 109
Pepsi® Twist 109
Persimmon, fresh 160
Pho soup (Vietnamese soup) 140
Picante taco sauce 149
Pickled beef 143
Pickled beets 166
Pillsbury® Big White Chunk Macadamia Nut Cookies 132
Pillsbury® Cinnamon Roll with Icing, all flavors 132
Pina colada 98
Pine nuts, pignolias 126
Pineapple juice 106
Pineapple orange drink 106
Pineapple, dried 160
Pineapple, fresh 160
Pistachio nuts, raw 126

Pizza Hut® cheese bread stick 140
Pizza Hut® Pepperoni Lover's pizza, stuffed crust 140
Pizza Hut® Personal Pan, supreme 140
Pizza, homemade or restaurant, cheese, thin crust 140
Plain dumplings for stew, biscuit type 146
Plantains, green, boiled 160
Plum, fresh 160
Polenta 147
Pomegranate juice 106
Pomegranate, fresh (arils-seed/juice sacs) 160
Poore Brothers® Potato Chips, Salt & Cracked Pepper 126
Popcorn, store bought (prepopped), "buttered" 132
Popsicle 171
Popsicle, sugar free 171

Pork cutlet, visible fat eaten 143
Port wine 98
Portabella mushrooms 166
Potato bread 111
Potato chips, salted 126
Potato dumpling (Kartoffelkloesse) 147
Potato gnocchi 147
Potato pancakes 147
Potato salad, with egg, mayo dressing 140
Potato soup with broccoli and cheese 140
Potato sticks 127
Potato, boiled, with skin 147
Potato, boiled, without skin 147
Power Bar® 20g Protein Plus, Chocolate Crisp 93
Power Bar® 20g Protein Plus, Chocolate Peanut Butter 93
Power Bar® 30g Protein Plus, Chocolate Brownie 94

Power Bar® Harvest Energy®, Double Chocolate Crisp 94
Power Bar® Performance Energy® 94
Powerade®, all flavors 94
Pretzels, hard, unsalted, sticks 127
Pringles® Light Fat Free Potato Crisps, Barbecue 127
Pringles® Potato Crisps, Loaded Baked Potato 127
Pringles® Potato Crisps, Original 127
Pringles® Potato Crisps, Salt & Vinegar 127
Pudding mix, other flavors, cooked type 122
Pumpernickel roll 111
Pumpkin or squash seeds 127
Purslane, raw 166

**Q**
Quince, fresh 160
Quinoa 147

**R**
Radicchio, raw 166
Radish, raw 166
Raisins, uncooked 160
Rambutan, canned in syrup 160
Ranch Crispy Chicken Wrap 149
Ranch salad dressing 154
Raspberries, fresh, red 160
Raspberry juice 107
Ratatouille 140
Red beans and rice soup mix, dry 140
Red Bull® Energy Drink 110
Red Bull® Energy Drink Sugar Free 110
Rhubarb pie, bottom crust only 132
Rhubarb, fresh 160
Ribs, beef, spare, visible fat eaten 143
Rice bread 111
Rice cake 127
Rice Krispies® (Kellogg's®) 115

Rice milk 122
Rice noodles, fried 147
Rice pudding (arroz con leche), coconut, raisins 122
Rice pudding (arroz con leche), plain 122
Rice pudding (arroz con leche), raisins 122
Ricotta cheese, part skim milk 123
Riesen® 135
Riesling 98
Ritz Cracker (Nabisco®) 127
Roast Beef Sandwich with Veggies, no mayo 154
Rob Roy 98
Rockstar Original® 110
Rockstar Original® Sugar Free 110
Rompope (eggnog with alcohol) 98
Root beer 98
Roquefort cheese 118
Rose hips 160
Rose wine, other types 98
Rum 98

Rum and cola 98
Rusty nail 98
Rutabaga, raw or blanched, marinated in oil mixture 166
Rye bread 111
Rye flour, in recipes not containing yeast 172
Rye roll 111

**S**
Sake 99
Salami, beer or beerwurst, beef 143
Salmon, red (sockeye), smoked 143
Sambuca 99
Sandwich cookies, vanilla 132
Sangria 99
Santa Claus melon 160
Sapodilla, fresh 160
Sauerbraten 144
Sauerkraut 167
Scallop squash 167
Scallops 144
Schnapps, all flavors 99
Schweppes® Bitter Lemon 110
Scotch and soda 99

Scrambled egg, made with bacon 140

Screwdriver 99

Sea Pak® Seasoned Shrimp, Roasted Garlic 144

Sea Pak® Shrimp Scampi in Parmesan Sauce 144

Seabreeze 99

Semolina flour 172

Sesame chicken 140

Sesame sticks 127

Shake, chocolate 149

Shake, strawberry 149

Shake, vanilla or other 149

Shallot, raw 167

Shiitake mushrooms, cooked 167

Singapore sling 99

Slim-Fast® Easy to Digest, Vanilla, ready-to-drink can 123

Sloe gin 99

Sloe gin fizz 99

Smart Balance® Light with Flax Oil Margarine, tub 118

Smart Balance® Margarine 118

Smarties® 135

Snickers® 135

Snickers®, Almond 135

Snow peas, cooked 167

Sorbet, chocolate 171

Sorbet, coconut 171

Sorbet, fruit 171

Sorghum 115

Souffle, meat 145

Soup base 140

Sour cherries, fresh 160

Sour cream 123

Sour pickles 167

Sourdough bread 111

Soursop (guanabana), fresh 161

Southern Comfort® 99

Soy bread 112

Soy chips 127

Soy Kaas Fat Free, all flavors 119

Soy milk, chocolate, sweetened with sugar, not fortified 103

Soy milk, plain or original, with artificial sweetener, ready 123

Soy milk, vanilla or other flavors, sugar, fat free, ready 123

Soybean sprouts, raw 167

Soybeans, cooked from dried 167

Spaetzle (spatzen) 147

Spaghetti squash 167

Spaghetti, with carbonara sauce 140

Spearmint tea 110

Special K® Blueberry cereal (Kellogg's®) 115

Special K® Cinnamon Pecan cereal (Kellogg's®) 115

Special K® Original cereal (Kellogg's®) 115

Special K® Red Berries cereal (Kellogg's®) 115

Spelt flour 172

Spiced ham loaf, canned 144

Spicy Italian Sandwich with Veggies, no meat 154

Spinach ravioli, with tomato sauce 140

Spinach, cooked from fresh 167

Splenda® 103

Split pea sprouts, cooked 167

Spring roll 140

Sprinkles Cookie Crisp® (General Mills®) 115

Sprite® 110

Sprite® Zero 110

Squash ravioli, with sauce 140

Starbucks® Hot Cocoa Double Chocolate 103

Starbucks® Hot Cocoa Salted Caramel, prepared 103

Starburst®, Original 136

Steak & Cheese Sandwich with Veggies 154

Stewed green peas & sofrito 141

Sticky bun 132

Stonyfield® Oikos Greek Yogurt, Blueberry 123

Stonyfield® Oikos Greek Yogurt, Caramel 123

Stonyfield® Oikos Greek Yogurt, Chocolate 123

Stonyfield® Oikos Greek Yo-gurt, Strawberry 123

Straw mushrooms, canned, drained 167

Strawberries, fresh 161

Strawberry milk, prepared 123

Strawberry pie, bottom crust only 132

Strawberry Shake 156

Streusel topping, crumb 172

Suckers®, sugar free 136

Sugar cookies, iced, store bought 132

Sugar, white granulated 136

Summer squash, cooked 167

Sunbelt Bakery® Granola Bar, Banana Harvest 115

Sunbelt Bakery® Chewy Granola Bar, Blueberry Harvest 115

Sunbelt Bakery® Chewy Granola Bar, Golden Almond 115

Sunbelt Bakery® Granola Bar, Low Fat Oatmeal Raisin 115

Sunbelt Bakery® Chewy Granola Bar, Oats & Honey 115

Sunbelt Bakery® Fudge Dipped Chewy Granola Bar, Coconut 115

Sundaes®, caramel 149

Sundaes®, chocolate fudge 149

Sundaes®, mini M & M® 149

Sundaes®, Oreo® 149

Sundaes®, strawberry 149

Sun-dried tomatoes, oil pack 167

Sunflower seeds, raw 127

Sushi, with fish 141

Sushi, with fish and vegetables in seaweed 141

Sushi, with vegetables 141

Swedish Meatballs 141

Sweet and sour chicken 141

Sweet and sour sauce 150

Sweet cherries, fresh 161

Sweet corn 150

Sweet Onion Chicken Teriyaki Sandwich with Veggies, no mayo 154

Sweet onion salad dressing 154

Sweet potato bread 132

Sweet potato, boiled 167

Sweetened condensed milk 103

Sweetened condensed milk, reduced fat 123

Swiss cheese, natural 119

Swiss cheese 119

Swiss Miss® Hot Cocoa Sensible Sweets Diet, sugar free, prepared 104

Sylvaner 99

**T**

Taco Bell® 7-Layer Burrito 141

Taco Bell® Beef Enchirito 155

Taco Bell® Caramel Apple Empanada 155

Taco Bell® Cheesy Fiesta Potatos 155

Taco Bell® cheesy gordita crunch 155

Taco Bell® Cinnamon Twists 155

Taco Bell® Combo Burrito 155

Taco Bell® Crunchwrap Supreme 141

Taco Bell® Double Decker Taco Supreme®, beef 155

Taco Bell® Mexican Pizza 141

Taco Bell® Nachos Supreme 141

Taco Bell® Pintos 'n Cheese 155

Taco John's® nachos 127

Taco with beans, cheese 141

Taffy 136

Tap water 110

Tempeh 167

TenderCrisp® Chicken Sandwich 149

Tequila 99

Tequila sunrise 99

Tic Tacs® 136

Tilsit cheese 119
Tiramisu 132
Toast, cinnamon and sugar, whole wheat bread 112
Toast, butter 112
Toblerone® Swiss Dark Chocolate with Honey & Almond Nougat 136
Toblerone® Swiss Milk Chocolate with Honey & Almond Nougat 136
Toblerone® Swiss White Confection with Honey & Almond Nougat 136
Toffee 136
Toffifay® 136
Tofu, raw (not silken), cooked, low fat 123
Tokaji Wine 99
Tomato juice 107
Tomato relish 141
Tomato soup mix, dry 141
Tomato, cooked from fresh 168
Tonic water 110
Tonic water, diet 110
Tootsie Pops® 136

Tortilla 127
Triple Sec 100
Triticale bread 112
Tuna Sandwich with Veggies, no mayo 154
Tuna 144
Turkey Breast & Ham Sandwich with Veggies 154
Turkey Breast Sandwich with Veggies 154
Turnip 168
Twix® 132

**V**
V-8® 100% A-C-E Vegetable Juice 107
Vanilla Coke® 110
Vegetable soup, condensed 141
Veggie Delite Salad 154
Veggie Delite Sandwich 154
Venison or deer, stewed 144
Veryfine Cranberry Raspberry 107
Vichyssoise 141
Vinegar 154
Vodka 100

**W**
Waffles, bran 132
Waffles mix 132
Walnuts 127
Watermelon, fresh 161
Wax beans 168
Weetabix® Organic Crispy 115
Wendys' 156
Werther's® Original Caramel Coffee Hard Candies 136
Wheat bran 172
Wheaties® 115
Whipped cream 104
Whipped cream, chocolate 123
Whipped cream, fat free 123
Whiskey 100
Whiskey sour 100
White flour 172
White bean stew with sofrito 141
White bread 112
White chip macadamia nut cookie 154
White chocolate Bar 136
White Russian 100
White tea 104
White whole grain wheat bread 112

White whole wheat flour 172
Whole wheat bread 112
Whopper® with cheese 149
Wild 'n Fruity Gummi Bears (Brach's®) 136
Windmill cookies 132
Wine spritzer 100
Winter melon 168
Winter type squash 168
Wise Onion Flavored Rings 127
Wrap bread 154

**Y**
Yams, sweet potato type 168
Yellow bell pepper, raw 168
Yellow tomato, raw 168
Yerba® Mate tea 110
Yogurt with aspartame 124
Yogurt with sucralose 124
Yogurt, fruited, whole milk 124

**Z**
Zesty onion ring sauce 149
Zsweet® 136

Made in United States
Orlando, FL
16 January 2022

13541614R00135